Lyme Disease

Lyme Disease

The Ecology of a Complex System

RICHARD S. OSTFELD

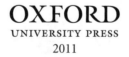
OXFORD
UNIVERSITY PRESS
2011

OXFORD

UNIVERSITY PRESS

Oxford University Press, Inc., publishes works that further
Oxford University's objective of excellence
in research, scholarship, and education.

Oxford   New York
Auckland   Cape Town   Dar es Salaam   Hong Kong   Karachi
Kuala Lumpur   Madrid   Melbourne   Mexico City   Nairobi
New Delhi   Shanghai   Taipei   Toronto

With offices in
Argentina   Austria   Brazil   Chile   Czech Republic   France   Greece
Guatemala   Hungary   Italy   Japan   Poland   Portugal   Singapore
South Korea   Switzerland   Thailand   Turkey   Ukraine   Vietnam

Copyright © 2011 by Oxford University Press, Inc.

Published by Oxford University Press, Inc.
198 Madison Avenue, New York, New York 10016

www.oup.com

Oxford is a registered trademark of Oxford University Press

Library of Congress Cataloging-in-Publication Data
Ostfeld, Richard S., 1954–
Lyme disease : the ecology of a complex system / Richard S. Ostfeld.
p. ; cm.
Includes bibliographical references and index.
ISBN 978-0-19-538812-1
1. Lyme disease—Environmental aspects. 2. Lyme disease—Epidemiology.
I. Title.
[DNLM: 1. Lyme Disease—epidemiology. 2. Arachnid Vectors.
3. Ecosystem. 4. Lyme Disease—transmission. 5. Risk Factors. WC 406 O85e 2010]
RA644.L94O88 2010
614.5'746—dc22   2010000805

1 3 5 7 9 8 6 4 2

Printed in the United States of America
on acid-free paper

For Felicia

Contents

Preface

GRADUATE STUDENTS GENERALLY SOCIALIZE WITH OTHER ACADEMICS and feel less comfortable hobnobbing in broader social strata. So I was mildly distressed to find myself at a cocktail party in 1985 faced with making conversation with a group of unfamiliar nonscientists. To get the ball rolling, I asked members of the circle what they did for a living. I learned that my small social group consisted of a marketer for a winery, an attorney, and an insurance broker. Their professions elicited no particular reaction from the others. But when I reported that I was a biologist, I was peppered with questions about what I really do. Pleased with the attention, I began to describe the wonders of studying animals in their natural habitats, only to be confronted by the insurance salesman with the question: But what does that contribute to society? My initial (silent) response was: Well, at least I don't convince people to buy things they don't really need. But I realized that the real challenge was to pithily describe to nonscientists why the pursuit of basic knowledge is worthwhile. I don't recall exactly how I answered, but my impression was that I did a poor job convincing these folks that knowing how nature works provides any tangible benefits to their lives. At the time, I was working on the territorial behavior of a rodent called the California vole (*Microtus californicus*), and perhaps its importance was a hard sell. Ever since that evening, I've felt that I need to be equipped to describe to any audience—scientific or not—why my science is important. If I fail to do so, perhaps the problem is not having an impenetrably dense audience, but rather having an insufficiently compelling research specialty.

The purpose of this book is to describe my understanding, based on the past 30 years of work by many excellent researchers, of where in nature Lyme disease comes from. What increases Lyme disease risk, what decreases it, why are there hotspots and bad years, and why is it spreading? The book is all about biology, from the spirochete bacterium (*Borrelia burgdorferi*) that causes the disease, to the tick vector, to the many animals ticks feed on, their habitats, the climate, the landscape, and beyond. So the natural audience for this book consists of ecologists, entomologists, epidemiologists, public health specialists, and students of all these disciplines. But I have tried to write the book so that nonscientists can follow the arguments. Perhaps I'm still trying to answer the insurance salesman. If he is among the many millions of people who live in the areas hard hit by this disease or is among the hundreds of thousands of past and current sufferers, perhaps he will be motivated to learn more about its ecology. This book will not give society a complete prescription for how to avoid or prevent Lyme disease, but there is practical information for those looking to reduce their odds of encountering an infected tick. One of the main points for nonbiologist readers, though, is that research in the science of ecology is useful for a variety of reasons, including helping protect human health.

My parents tell me that as a child I had a habit of being contrarian. The famous family story (and I would wager it's apocryphal) is that, as I was putting on my jacket to go outside for an afternoon of playing ball, my mother said: Have a good time, to which I reportedly responded: Don't tell me what to do. Regardless of this particular story's veracity, I admit to being an iconoclast by nature. In 1991, about a year into my current academic position at the Cary Institute of Ecosystem Studies in Millbrook, New York, I began a new field research project that involved studying populations of white-footed mice (*Peromyscus leucopus*). I was collaborating with my new colleagues Charles Canham, Clive Jones, and Gary Lovett in asking whether mice could prevent a forest pest, the gypsy moth (*Lymantria dispar*), from undergoing outbreaks and killing millions of trees. So initially this research had nothing to do with Lyme disease.

Field research on mice typically involves trapping them in small metal box traps and then inspecting and marking them before letting them go. The mice at the Cary Institute were typical of the many thousands of other rodents I had previously trapped except for one feature—their ears were covered with the ticks responsible for transmitting the Lyme disease bacterium. Thus began my interest in Lyme disease ecology. Small rodents like mice were notorious for undergoing boom and bust cycles, and many scientists were researching the causes of these fluctuations. I decided to ask what the *consequences* of those fluctuations might be for tick populations and Lyme disease risk.

To undertake a new research project in an unfamiliar area, a scientist needs to start by reading the pertinent literature. In doing so, I was impressed by how much of the ecology of Lyme disease had been worked out in the 15 or so years since the disease was first discovered. But the picture that this literature painted of Lyme disease ecology seemed much too simple. It focused on only a small subset of the species that ticks feed on, and it was limited to few habitats, processes, and seasons. As I continued with my research on mice, deer, other vertebrates, ticks, spirochetes, and their habitats, the data my group collected were often inconsistent with the concepts advocated by prior research. The discrepancies are described in detail in the chapters that follow; suffice it to say that my iconoclastic nature led me to question the dogma that permeated the literature. Of course, questioning paradigms is only a part of the scientific process—to advance our knowledge, one must contribute to the replacement of prior views with new understanding. That is what I have tried to do in my research, and what I try to do in this book.

The ideas and information in this book arose from many sources. In acknowledging the importance of interactions with colleagues, students, and others, I wish to recognize their impacts on my thinking while taking full responsibility for the arguments in this book. Indeed, it's safe to say that many who have influenced me do not agree with my understanding of the evidence. Discussions with Lyme disease pioneers Durland Fish, Joe Piesman, Mark Wilson, Tom Mather, and Howard Ginsberg early in my work in this complex disease system strongly influenced my thinking. Colleagues at the Cary Institute, particularly Charlie Canham, Alan Berkowitz, and Mike Pace, have been consistently generous with their thoughts and technical skills and have listened to me blather. Former graduate students and postdocs in my lab, especially Josh Van Buskirk, Ken Schmidt, Kathleen LoGiudice, Eric Schauber, Brian Allan, Jesse Brunner, Dustin Brisson, Lisa Schwanz, Andrea Previtali, and Mary Killilea, contributed to the generation of many of the ideas in this book and to my general education as a scientist. Research specialists Kelly Oggenfuss, Shannon Duerr, Buck West, Chris Neil, Deanna Sloniker, and Holly Vuong and the dozens of project assistants that worked with them over the years are responsible for generating most of the data described herein. Matt Gillespie and Lynn Sticker worked their usual magic with figures, references, and other technical issues. Ray Winchcombe facilitated my use of ideal research sites at the Cary Institute, and many home owners, schools, and businesses in

New York, Connecticut, and New Jersey generously allowed my research team access to their properties to do our research. Amy Schuler acquired interlibrary loan papers at light speed. Marie Smith and Kate Wallen provided much logistic support in grant proposals and administration. Bill Schlesinger granted me a semester's leave to make headway in writing this book. Many other people at the Cary Institute deserve credit for making it the most stimulating and supportive professional environment I can imagine.

Funding for my laboratory's research on Lyme disease has been generously provided by the National Science Foundation, the National Institutes of Health, the U.S. Environmental Protection Agency, the Centers for Disease Control and Prevention, Dutchess County, New York, and its taxpayers and government, the Nathan Cummings Foundation, the Plymouth Hill Foundation, the General Reinsurance Corporation, and the Andrew W. Mellon Foundation. A grant from the Opportunities for Providing Understanding through Synthesis (OPUS) program of the National Science Foundation was instrumental in providing the time and resources to write the manuscript. Without the OPUS program, I would not have written this book.

I am deeply grateful to Leon Botstein, Michèle Dominy, Mark Halsey, Mike Tibbetts, Philip Johns, Meghan Karcher, and Mike Rich, all from Bard College, for their support and hospitality during my leave there in winter and spring of 2009 when I did most of the writing. My office in the Reem-Kayden Center was the perfect place to think and write. My editors at Oxford University Press, Phyllis Cohen and Peter Prescott, provided essential advice, encouragement, and technical support throughout the process. Graeme Cumming and his students and Janet Sperling read and provided helpful comments on the manuscript.

My parents, Ruth and Adrian Ostfeld, created a home environment in which independence of thought was valued and nurtured, even when it led to near self-destruction.

Most of the concepts explored in this book were developed in collaboration with my wife and colleague, Felicia Keesing. She also read the entire manuscript, providing invaluable input big and small. Without her insight, creativity, guidance, and partnership, there would have been no book to write. She can chase kori bustards, potty train children, and cook up 20-minute meals with equal skill. My gratitude can't be expressed.

Lyme Disease

1

Introduction

LYME DISEASE IS NOTHING IF NOT CONTROVERSIAL. PITCHED BATTLES have been raging for years between two diametrically opposed views of how common it is, how easy it is to diagnose and treat, how to treat it, and whether it exists in a chronic form. The disagreements have led to an unfortunate situation in which proponents of the opposing views distrust each other, even to the point of impugning each other's motives and integrity.

On the one hand are groups of patients and some practicing physicians who assert that Lyme disease is vastly more common and more severe than indicated by most statistics, that most cases are unrecognized and undiagnosed, and that this leads to inadequate treatment (or none at all) with the result that many patients become chronically infected. The biomedical research community is seen as largely responsible for failing to recognize the size of the problem, which leads to inadequate attention to diagnostic tools and effective treatments. Insurance companies, which benefit from strictly limiting the tests and treatments that are covered under policies, are viewed as complicit or even pulling the strings of physician-puppets. Patient health is a casualty of stubborn adherence to a world view unsupported by evidence and guided by financial motives.

On the other hand are groups of researchers and physicians who argue that Lyme disease is relatively difficult to contract and easy to treat with oral antibiotic therapy. They are concerned that symptoms and syndromes unrelated to Lyme disease are frequently misdiagnosed as Lyme disease and that the treatments often prescribed are both ineffective and potentially dangerous to patients. Patient-advocates and some physicians who treat them are seen as ill informed and out of the mainstream. They sometimes accuse these patients of paranoia and hypochondria and the physicians willing to treat them with intravenous antibiotics and other radical measures as guilty of poor practice or even malpractice.

Patient-advocates and biomedical researchers have clashed over detections of and responses to other diseases, but the animosity between these two groups in the case of Lyme disease seems extreme in both its depth and duration. The attorney general of the State of Connecticut recently threatened to sue the Infectious Diseases Society of America (IDSA), stating in a May 1, 2008, press release, "The IDSA's guideline panel improperly ignored or minimized consideration of alternative medical opinion and evidence regarding chronic Lyme disease, potentially raising serious questions about whether the recommendations reflected all relevant science." The IDSA was forced to convene a special panel that spent more than a year reviewing evidence pertaining to guidelines on diagnosis and treatment of Lyme disease. (The review panel unanimously upheld the IDSA guidelines, but this is unlikely to dampen the controversy.) In February of 2009, Congressman Chris Smith (R-NJ) introduced the "Lyme and Tick-Borne Disease Prevention, Education, and Research Act of 2009" (H.R. 1179), which would spend $100 million over five years to expand federal efforts concerning the prevention, education, treatment, and research activities related to Lyme and other tick-borne diseases. One would think that a dramatic increase in federal funding on Lyme disease would be a point of strong agreement between the two opposing groups, but one would be wrong. H.R. 1179 stipulates that allocation of funds would be guided by a Tick-Borne Diseases Advisory Committee, which must consist of the following

i. At least 4 members from the scientific community representing the broad spectrum of viewpoints held within the scientific community related to Lyme and other tick-borne diseases.
ii. At least 2 representatives of tick-borne disease voluntary organizations.
iii. At least 2 health care providers, including at least 1 full-time practicing physician, with relevant experience providing care for individuals with a broad range of acute and chronic tick-borne diseases.
iv. At least 2 patient representatives who are individuals who have been diagnosed with a tick-borne disease or who have had an immediate family member diagnosed with such a disease, and
v. At least 2 representatives of State and local health departments and national organizations that represent State and local health professionals.

Voices in the biomedical research community adamantly oppose what they see as an attempt to dilute or distort mainstream views with those that would be represented by this list and are vociferously urging "no" votes in Congress. No obvious signs indicate that this controversy will abate any time soon.

Why diagnosis and treatment for Lyme disease are so much more contentious than for other diseases is not clear. I suspect that one key reason is that the causative agent—the spirochete bacterium *Borrelia burgdorferi*—is a uniquely complicated pathogen that presents unusually difficult challenges. If we knew which patients were actually infected and for how long, then at least some of the controversy would disappear. But the diagnostic tests are relatively poor and behave in frustrating ways—both positive and negative test results can be wrong. This leads to the misidentification of people with Lyme disease as uninfected and of uninfected people as having Lyme disease. Poor diagnostic accuracy for Lyme disease contrasts starkly with those of most other infectious diseases we commonly experience. And the consequences of misdiagnosis are often more critical for Lyme disease than for other diseases. This is because, in contrast to many other infections, our immune systems are shockingly poor at curing us of Lyme disease, leading to potentially severe disease if antibiotics are not used. On the other hand, overuse of antibiotics in patients not needing them can be strongly detrimental to the patient and can also increase the evolution of antibiotic resistance by various microbes. The lack of reliable diagnostic tests, combined with the lack of a vaccine, means that health care providers are unusually impotent in protecting and curing patients, and much of the health care burden shifts to patients and potential patients. The controversy itself seems to further increase the feelings of isolation and self-responsibility among patients.

The fact that people are forced to be largely self-reliant in dealing with the threat or occurrence of Lyme disease means that information on how to avoid exposure becomes all the more imperative. We know that exposure to *B. burgdorferi* bacteria can only occur through the bite of a particular type of tick (a possible exception is rare transplacental transmission). The main culprit in most of North America is the blacklegged tick, *Ixodes scapularis*. That aspect of Lyme disease epidemiology is uncontroversial. But simply knowing that Lyme bacteria come from ticks is hardly adequate to offer any real protection. Instead, we need to know *where* ticks are most abundant and why, *when* ticks are most abundant and why, and *where* and *when* ticks are most heavily infected with *B. burgdorferi*. The *where* and *when* parts would allow us to avoid exposure to ticks or, if avoidance is impractical, to target tick control efforts at the places and times of greatest risk. And if we knew *why* ticks were abundant and heavily infected here but not there, and now but not then, we would have the information necessary to manage habitats or landscapes to reduce risk, in environmentally sensitive ways. So, avoidance and management of Lyme disease require an understanding of the factors that determine the distribution and abundance of some specific organisms involved in the maintenance and transmission of Lyme disease in nature. The scientific discipline devoted to understanding the distribution and abundance of organisms is called *ecology*.

Ecology is rarely thought of by nonecologists as an integral part of the health sciences. But a moment's thought about what constitutes an infectious disease reveals that ecology is fundamentally important. The simplest of infectious disease systems involves two organisms—the pathogen and its host. The host's risk of being exposed to the pathogen is fundamentally a consequence of the distribution and abundance of both organisms and how they interact. So, even the common cold is an ecological system composed of two organisms—the virus and the human host—co-occupying a habitat, typically a house, school, or office. Sometimes the interactions giving rise to a new case of the cold are obvious, for example, when a child sneezes millions of rhinovirus particles into his mother's face. Other times the causes of exposure are somewhat more complex, for example, when a college professor rubs her runny nose and seconds later grabs a door handle, which is then grasped by several students entering the classroom. Perhaps the professor is the same mother who was anointed with the sneeze two days earlier and is shedding virus particles despite not yet feeling sick. Or perhaps she returned to her American college recently from a trip to Europe, where she shook hands with a colleague who was harboring a strain of rhinovirus that had not yet penetrated the Western hemisphere. If she had had the opportunity to wash her hands after meeting the colleague, she might have returned home pathogen-free.

These scenarios provide examples of how distinctly ecological this cold system is. The pathogen has multiple means of dispersing short distances but can also disperse long distances. The social behavior, self-grooming habits, and local population density of the host are important to transmission. The pathogen is subject to evolutionary change (mutation and natural selection) that influences its interactions with predators (in this case, the host's antibodies). It undergoes population growth and decline within a host that determines its likelihood of emigrating from that host and immigrating to others. Any infectious disease is inherently an ecological system.

The Lyme disease system is much more complex than the common cold, and many of its complexities involve the addition of more species and habitats in which ecological interactions occur. Lyme disease is a *zoonosis*, meaning that the pathogen typically resides in one or more non-human vertebrate hosts from which it can be transmitted to humans. These vertebrates that maintain and amplify the pathogen in nature—and thus become the source of infection when it spreads to other hosts—are called *reservoirs*. Lyme disease is also a *vector-borne* disease, meaning that the pathogen moves from one host to another during the bite of a blood-feeding arthropod (in this case, a tick). So, we've now added at least two new species—a tick vector and a reservoir for the pathogen—to the simple pathogen–human system. Because each of these two new species has complex ecological interactions of its own, the degree of system complexity has risen exponentially. And, what if there are several species of vertebrates that can act as reservoirs? What if there is more than one vector? What if these reservoir species interact with one another, either directly (for instance, by competing for the same food) or indirectly (for example, by attracting ticks that might have fed on another species)? The ecological complexity of the system can quickly become daunting (figure 1).

The tendency among biomedical researchers who specialize in diseases that are zoonotic or vector-borne, or both, is to pare down the ecological world to the smallest group of species and interactions thought to be critical in maintaining and transmitting the pathogen. They tend to seek "the" reservoir, "the" vector, "the" habitat, responsible for disease. This approach arises from the dominant *reductionist* paradigm of biomedicine, which seeks to understand phenomena by pursuing simpler, smaller, or more proximate levels of organization. Reductionism in biomedicine has been a phenomenally successful approach, yet for some issues it is inadequate. Understanding the ecological determinants of infectious disease risk is one of those issues. Unfortunately, ecological science, which includes both reductionist and holistic approaches, has a bad rap both among practitioners of other scientific disciplines and among some elements of the lay public. When it's not being confused with environmentalism, ecology is typically thought of as a "soft" science that's too holistic and squishy to play a reliable role in public health. An anecdote might help explain how nonecologist scientists view ecological science, and why they might not want to depend on it for their health.

Just as I began my research into the ecology of Lyme disease in 1991, I read what to me was an astonishing statement by leading scientists about ecological systems. The statement was published in *Science* magazine as a

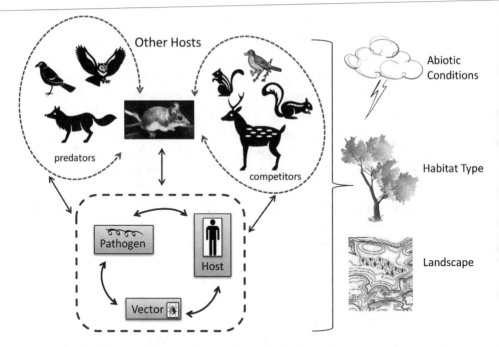

FIGURE 1. Diagram of the complexity inherent in the Lyme disease system in most of North America. At the heart of the disease system are the interactions between the pathogen (*Borrelia burgdorferi*), the vector (*Ixodes scapularis*), and human victims. Some hosts for ticks, such as white-footed mice (*Peromyscus leucopus*), play important roles in transmitting pathogens to ticks during blood meals. Many other vertebrates that inhabit these ecological communities play multiple roles, including attracting ticks away from mice and preying on or competing with mice. These ecological interactions, described in later chapters of this book, occur within a context of variable and changing climate, variable habitat quality for all the animals involved, and differing landscapes.

part of what was called the "Top 20 Greatest Hits of Science" (figure 2). This was a list of the 20 most important, fundamental, and enduring generalities, or "laws," in all of the sciences; it was intended to provide focus for efforts at increasing scientific literacy among nonscientists. The list had entries that covered the laws of thermodynamics, the genetic code embodied in nucleic acids, the shifting positions of continental plates (continental drift), the evolution of life forms by natural selection, the origin of the universe in the Big Bang, and others. The science of ecology was represented by one entry, listed as number 20: "All life is connected."

Of course, this statement in no way represents a universal law of ecology and does not belong in a list intended to foster scientific literacy. The main reason is that it's too vague to interpret unequivocally or to evaluate rigorously. What is meant by "life" in this context? Do we mean that

Science's Top 20 Greatest Hits

1. **The universe is regular and predictable.**
   The next six overarching principles underlie all the rest of science, beginning with Newton's three laws of motion, which are summarized by:

2. **One set of laws describes all motion.**
   The First and Second Laws of Thermodynamics govern the behavior of heat and energy:

3. **Energy is conserved;** and

4. **Energy always goes from more useful to less useful forms.**
   Everything we know about electricity, magnetism, and electromagnetic radiation, which includes visible light, infrared and ultraviolet radiation, microwaves, x-rays, and radiowaves, starts with the realization that:

5. **Electricity and magnetism are two aspects of the same force.**
   The fundamental nature of matter and energy is summed up by two more great ideas:

6. **Everything is made of atoms;** and

7. **Everything -- particles energy, the rate of electron spin – comes in discrete units, and you can't measure anything without changing it.**
   Next, the different basic fields of science and the fundamental ideas underlying each are identified, starting with chemistry:

8. **Atoms are bound together by electron "glue";** and

9. **The way a material behaves depends on how its atoms are arranged.**
   Five great ideas in physics, ranging from fundamental particls to astrophysics and cosmology:

10. **Nuclear energy comes from the conversion of mass;**

11. **Everything is really made of quarks and leptons;**

12. **Stars live and die like everything else;**

13. **The universe was born at a specific time in the past, and it has been expanding ever since;** and

14. **Every observer sees the same laws of nature** (a summation of Einstein's special and general theories of relativity). Modern geology, geophysics and earth sciences rest on the understanding that:

15. **The surface of the earth is constantly changing, and no feature on the earth is permanent;** and

16. **Everything on the earth operates in cycles.**
    And to comprehend biology, the study of life on earth, one needs to know that:

17. **All living things are made of cells, the chemical factories of life;**

18. **All life is based on the same genetic code;**

19. **All forms of life evolved by natural selection;** and

20. **All life is connected.**

FIGURE 2. "Science's Top 20 Greatest Hits,." This list was meant to represent the most important, overarching generalities in all of the sciences. Note that the discipline of ecology is addressed with number 20 on the list. *Source:* Adapted from Pool (1991).

all life forms, or species, are connected? And what is meant by "connected"? Do we mean that if one species is somehow disturbed or changed in some way, then all other species on the planet will respond in some detectable way? All the other entries in the Top 20 Greatest Hits can be, and have been, rigorously tested and evaluated, and decades or centuries of research have found them to be robust. "All life is connected" is either a false statement (think about trying to detect an effect of an oak tree falling in Delaware on a blue whale in the South Pacific) or utterly untestable. Yet, this represents the fundamental truth of ecological science to other scientists! Clearly, a similar view of ecology also pervades the lay public (when they think about ecology at all). How often do we hear people utter (or utter ourselves) something to the effect that "everything is connected to everything else"? John Muir's statement in *My First Summer in the Sierra*, "When we try to pick out anything by itself, we find it hitched to everything else in the universe," is lovely poetry, but it is not science.

No wonder, then, that ecology might not generally be included the list of scientific disciplines considered crucial in understanding and combating health threats. But in the case of Lyme and many other diseases, we have no choice. These diseases exist only because of a complex set of interactions among many species off in nature that we are unwittingly exposed to when we venture forth. Various failed attempts to predict and control Lyme disease—described in later chapters—illustrate the limitations of a reductionist attempt to comprehend the complexity inherent to the system. Of course, it would not be productive to replace an overly reductionist, exclusionary focus with one that is too inclusive, holistic, and soft. What we need for understanding Lyme disease risk are rigorous models of the disease that include all the species, habitats, and processes that are essential, and nothing else.

So, this book is about one approach to understanding the dizzying complexity of an ecological system, but one that is pressured by considerable urgency, knowing that the health of millions of people is compromised or at risk. In a nutshell, this approach consists of a dialog between homing in (reductionism) and zooming out (holism), and integrating between them along the way. This is essentially the approach I have taken to the ecology of Lyme disease. Fundamentally, what we need to know is where and when we are most at risk, and why. We do have crude maps showing where Lyme disease is distributed in some regions of the world. We know that the onset of new cases peaks in summer. And we have lists of the habitats in which ticks occur, and the hosts they sometimes feed on. To some, this is enough ecological knowledge to paint a useful picture of where Lyme disease comes from. But this knowledge has not resulted in the development of interventions that might prevent Lyme disease from continuing to expand and increase in intensity. In my view, an overly simplistic view of Lyme disease ecology and risk, which developed largely from chance events (described in the coming chapters) combined with a reductionist tradition that pervades biomedical sciences, has led to a false sense of understanding.

In the chapters to follow I briefly describe the events leading to the discovery of what is now called Lyme disease, or Lyme borreliosis. This discussion indicates how the place where Lyme disease emerged in the United States set the stage for the basic ecological model of disease risk that largely persists to the present. The early investigations to identify the species involved in Lyme disease transmission were indeed impressive in their scope and pace, and much of the information gathered in the early years remains useful today. However, I also describe how some of this information led to the establishment of what I consider dogma that has resisted the incorporation of new knowledge. Our developing understanding of the ecology of Lyme disease can be seen as a parable for the pursuit of ecological knowledge more broadly. The more we understand, the more complex and inclusive our models of the system become. The urge to stop this creeping expansionism is strong, as we worry that clear conceptual models will be replaced by platitudes about connectedness. The challenge, then, is to embrace the complexity that is essential, identify components that are not, and maintain the clarity of models for how the system works.

Despite its complexity, risk of human exposure to Lyme disease is often predictable. We know that walking into a small woodlot is much riskier than walking into a nearby large, extensive forest. We know that hiking in the oak woods two summers after a big acorn year is much riskier than hiking in those same woods after an acorn failure. We know that forests that house many species of mammals and birds are safer than those that support fewer species. We know that the more opossums and squirrels there are in the woods, the lower the risk of Lyme disease, and we suspect that the same is true of owls, hawks, and weasels. And we know that year-to-year variation in climate has little effect on Lyme disease risk (although long-term climate change might). Before describing why forest size, biodiversity, acorns, and opossums are important and local climate seemingly is not, it's first necessary to describe the evolution of the major paradigm of Lyme disease ecology, namely, that the white-tailed deer is the main actor determining risk, with mice and climate playing supporting roles. This is the main topic of the next several chapters.

Before proceeding to describe the Lyme disease paradigm and its evolution, let me define the scope of the discussion. This book focuses on Lyme disease in eastern and central North America, where incidence rates are highest and controversy strongest. Lyme disease also occurs in far western North America and is a major public health concern in parts of Europe and Asia. Although many aspects of Lyme disease ecology in these other localities are strikingly similar to those in eastern and central North America, some others are not. Different tick species transmit the pathogen in western North America, Europe, and Asia, different genotypes of the *Borrelia* pathogen are present, and vertebrate host communities are quite variable across the globe. Although I suspect that ecological interactions in these other localities strongly parallel those in eastern/central North America, information for testing this hypothesis is often lacking.

2

Discovery

EMERGING INFECTIOUS DISEASES HAVE A HUGE IMPACT ON HUMAN societies, causing millions of deaths and untold suffering, while costing tens of billions of U.S. dollars annually. *Emerging infectious diseases* are defined as those infectious diseases that appear suddenly or increase dramatically in incidence or geographic extent. Some diseases known to have emerged previously but that have subsided can "reemerge." The appearance of such diseases can be caused by quite different phenomena. In the case of HIV/AIDS, disease emergence in humans in the 1970s and 1980s was caused by the recent mutation in an ape virus that allowed it to invade human bodies and to do so with devastating consequences to the victim. In the parlance of disease biology, the virus shifted its host range, or *host-jumped*, from apes to humans and increased in virulence. This emergence event was caused by the evolution of a "new" pathogen—one that was sufficiently genetically distinct to cause a new disease in a new host. In other cases, such as West Nile virus, disease emergence can be caused by a sudden expansion of a well-known pathogen into a new geographic area. The emergence of disease caused by West Nile virus occurred after the accidental introduction of the virus from the Middle East to the New York City area in 1999. Perhaps the most common mode by which diseases emerge is the sudden recognition of a disease that has been present for some time but that had existed under the biomedical radar. This is the mode by which Lyme disease emerged.

Lyme disease is not new. Symptoms that almost certainly represent cases of Lyme disease were described in the European medical literature in the late nineteenth century (Stanek et al. 2002). Molecular evidence of the presence of the bacterium that causes Lyme disease has been found in museum specimens of rodents that were collected in the early twentieth century (Sonenshine 1993). A resident of Lyme, Connecticut, named Polly Murray, who is credited with the original detective work that alerted biomedical experts that a new disease might exist, probably suffered from Lyme disease as early as the 1950s (Weintraub 2008).

A critical milestone in all disease emergences occurs when the causative agent is identified. Knowing what causes the illness allows biomedical scientists to develop or recommend methods to diagnose an infection and sometimes provide cures (for example, specific antimicrobial drugs). Such knowledge also is necessary for the development of preventive measures such as vaccines. But vaccine development is agonizingly slow and fraught with problems. Most of the diseases that have emerged in the past half-century, including Lyme disease, still have no widely available vaccine. Of course, vaccines are not the only preventive measure available to populations at risk of exposure to infectious diseases. To the extent that we can avoid infection with the disease agent in the first place, we will be able to prevent illness. Knowing how to avoid infection requires much more information than simply what microbe causes the disease.

Two additional key bits of information are where the microbe exists when it's not in a human body, and how it gets from that place to a person. For various emerging infectious diseases, the pathogens can reside in water, soil, air, food, or the bodily fluids of other people, and we get sick when we unwittingly drink, breathe, eat, or otherwise contact them. Preventing exposure to these pathogens can be aided by specific knowledge of what specific substrate is needed by the pathogen and where it's likely to multiply, or *replicate*. But for most emerging infectious diseases—up to 75% by some accounts (Taylor et al. 2001)—the pathogen dwells and replicates in the bodies of nonhuman, vertebrate animals such as rodents, bats, birds, or livestock. The diseases caused by these pathogens are called *zoonoses*. For zoonoses (also called *zoonotic diseases*), avoidance of human exposure to the disease agent requires that we identify the vertebrate species in which the pathogen resides and replicates—the *reservoirs*. This might seem to be a simple enough task, and indeed it can be simple when there is a single or very small number of reservoir species. However, most zoonotic diseases have several or even many reservoirs, and these reservoir species can differ dramatically in how long they can host the pathogen, how well the pathogen replicates inside them, and which genetic strains of the pathogen are best supported. These differences among vertebrates in what is called their *reservoir competence* exist because of species-specific variation in immune function. However, the specific aspects of the immune system that allow some species to prevent or quickly clear an infection and others to permit rampant replication by the pathogen are not well characterized for most zoonoses.

For some zoonoses, the mechanical means by which the pathogen gets from its reservoir host to the human victim is fairly direct. For example, the hantaviruses are a group of zoonotic pathogens that persist in rodents and can cause severe hemorrhaging, kidney disease, or lung disease in humans. The rodents are thought to infect one another during fights when an infected individual bites or scratches an uninfected one. The virus replicates within the newly infected rodent but does not appear to make the rodent host very sick, so the infected rodent goes about releasing virus particles by the millions in its urine and feces, often for weeks or even months. When the excreta dry, the virus particles can become airborne. Humans can get infected with hantavirus when they breathe these airborne bits of virus-contaminated rodent excreta. Each type of hantavirus tends to infect a specific species of rodent, so the hantaviruses provide examples of relatively simple systems for prescribing ecologically based prevention. Keeping those rodents out of human dwellings and avoiding places where they defecate and urinate are recommended.

For other zoonoses, however, the pathogen cannot persist outside of an animal's body, and the only means for them to travel from one vertebrate host to another is by hitching a ride inside another animal. These pathogens have evolved to take advantage of the blood-feeding habits of many arthropod species such as mosquitoes, fleas, and ticks, using the arthropod as a means of transportation from one vertebrate's circulatory system to another's. The diseases caused by these pathogens are called *vector-borne diseases*. The challenges facing a microbial pathogen's ability to adapt physiologically to such distinct environments as the gut of an arthropod and the bloodstream of a vertebrate would seem daunting. Apparently, however, the evolutionary benefits of such an efficient mode of dispersal from the circulatory system of one vertebrate host to that of another outweigh the costs of contending with such disparate environments.

The Black Death, or bubonic plague, that killed millions of Asians in the fourteenth century and millions more Europeans in the seventeenth century is perhaps the most infamous of the vector-borne zoonotic diseases. The bacterium that causes plague is *Yersinia pestis*, which replicates inside various species of rodents, including rats. This bacterium is particularly versatile in its means of moving from one host to another, sometimes dispersing via bodily fluids, but its preferred route is inside the guts of fleas. Flea species tend to strongly prefer a single species of host, but under some circumstances they will switch from their preferred host to others. When fleas have plenty of rodents to bite, or when the rodent hosts are physically separated from human habitations, then *Yersinia*-infected fleas bite humans only rarely. In these situations, risk of human disease is very low and the pathogen is said to persist in an *enzootic cycle*, that is, only among non-human animals. But when rodents live in close proximity to humans, opportunities arise for the fleas to switch from biting rodents to biting people, and disease risk can skyrocket. Of course, proximity of rodents to humans by itself is insufficient to cause an increase in human disease—it is also necessary that the fleas are interested in biting humans. Some arthropod vectors are extremely picky about which vertebrates they will bite, and these tend not to be important zoonotic vectors simply because they rarely bite humans. The vectors that are less selective in their choice of hosts—the *host-generalists*—are the ones that are most troublesome.

But simply knowing which hosts a particular vector species will bite—its *host range*—is inadequate for understanding disease risk. The fleas that transmit plague bacteria might normally restrict themselves to rat's nests, biting rats and only rats. Imagine what might happen, though, if the rat colony is eradicated one night by hungry cats, leaving a flea-infested rat's nest with no rats. If the rat's nest happens to be in the thatched roof of a London village house in the 1660s, the fleas might leave their roof nest seeking some other warm-blooded host, and find nothing but human cohabitants. This basic scenario is considered quite plausible in causing some of the major plague epidemics that struck prominent European cities several centuries ago. Either sudden or gradual changes in the relative availability of different host species, caused by changing ecological conditions, probably played a strong role in these devastating epidemics.

So what do we need to establish quickly if we want to understand why a new zoonotic disease emerged and what we can do to prevent it? The list of necessary bits of information has grown from simply the identity of the pathogen, to the identities of the vertebrate reservoirs, of which there might be several or even many, to the identity of the vector, to the host range of the vector, to the ecological conditions that might cause the vector to shift its host preferences. This set of information is difficult to obtain and can require decades of ecological detective work. But prescribing effective means of avoidance and prevention requires such knowledge.

The Beginnings of Lyme Disease

Juvenile rheumatoid arthritis (JRA) is a disease characterized by painful swelling of joints in children ranging in age from 6 months to 16 years. It appears to be an autoimmune disease caused by white blood cells attacking and damaging healthy tissues in and around the joints. What causes the immune system of JRA patients to attack their own tissues is not well understood. JRA is relatively rare, affecting only about 50,000 to 75,000 children in the United States. The odds of a rare disease like JRA affecting more than one or two children in a town of a few thousand inhabitants are vanishingly small. But in the mid-1970s, two residents of Lyme, Connecticut (population ~ 2000), Polly Murray and Judith Mensch, became concerned that not only their own children but also those of several neighbors had been diagnosed with JRA. Lyme is an affluent, exurban town situated a few kilometers from Long Island Sound in southern Connecticut. Murray and Mensch independently compiled notes on cases of arthritis in neighborhood children and contacted the Connecticut Department of Health in 1975, and both were referred to physician-researchers at Yale University.

When a relatively rare disease seems to occur in a cluster, suspicions arise that some localized cause is to blame. The per-capita incidence of painful joint swelling in children in and around Lyme was about 100 times greater than that of JRA in the general population, leading to reasonable certainty that in fact a cluster of disease cases had been identified. The most obvious culprits that could cause a geographically restricted disease outbreak are point-source contaminants and localized infectious agents. No further evidence supported the notion that some local environmental or food contaminant was to blame, so attention was turned to infectious agents. The Yale researchers, most notably Allen Steere, ascertained that many of the patients with JRA had experienced a skin rash several weeks before their joints became swollen and painful and hypothesized that the rash and arthritic conditions were linked by a common cause.

Researchers from Yale University began to monitor the health of patients following the appearance of similar skin lesions, finding that many of them later developed arthritis as well as nervous system and heart disorders. These researchers were aware of previously described co-occurrences of similar skin lesions (called *erythema migrans*) with joint pain and neuritis in the European medical literature from the late nineteenth century (figure 3). This European syndrome had been associated with tick bites, and although the causative agent had never been identified, many patients responded well to treatment with penicillin. This observation strongly suggested a bacterial cause (reviewed by Stanek et al. 2002). Yale researchers named the new disease Lyme disease, suspecting that it was caused by bacteria transmitted by ticks. However, neither the bacterium nor the possible vector had been identified by the end of the 1970s.

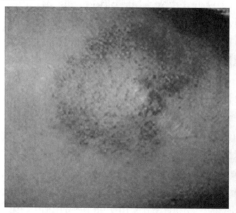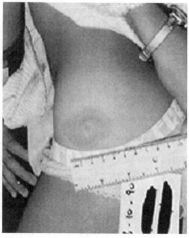

FIGURE 3. Erythema migrans, or bull's-eye rashes, of Lyme disease sufferers. These rashes are among the primary early symptoms used to diagnose Lyme disease. Other early symptoms of Lyme disease include fever, chills, muscle aches, headaches, and lethargy. If not treated early after the onset of symptoms, patients can later suffer from facial paralysis (Bell's palsy), various other neurological ailments, carditis, and arthritis.

Meanwhile, across Long Island Sound from Lyme, Connecticut, researchers Jorge Benach and Edward Bosler were undertaking ecological reconnaissance for the tick vectors of a well-known vector-borne zoonosis, Rocky Mountain spotted fever. This disease had killed as many as eight residents of Long Island, New York, in the late 1970s and early 1980s, and these biologists were surveying for the American dog tick, *Dermacentor variabilis,* which is the main vector of *Rickettsia rickettsii,* the causative agent of Rocky Mountain Spotted Fever. *Dermacentor* ticks were indeed present, but another tick species belonging to the genus *Ixodes* was much more locally abundant than were dog ticks. Benach and Bosler sent specimens of these *Ixodes* ticks to the laboratory of their collaborator Willy Burgdorfer, where the ticks were to be assayed for *Rickettsia* (figure 4). Burgdorfer did not find *Rickettsia* in the Long Island *Ixodes* ticks, but he did find that about 60% contained a spirochete bacterium of unknown identity in their midguts (Burgdorfer et al. 1982). Suspecting that they might have found the causative agent of Lyme disease, the researchers isolated and cultured the spirochetes. They found that the spirochetes caused clinical signs in laboratory animals consistent with symptoms of Lyme disease in humans, and they later determined that Lyme disease patients indeed were infected with these spirochetes (Burgdorfer et al. 1982, Benach et al. 1983). The group of researchers named the newly described bacterium *Borrelia burgdorferi* in honor of its key discoverer (Johnson et al. 1984) (figure 5).

The identity of the tick vector responsible for transmitting *B. burgdorferi* was very much in doubt at this time. Harvard researcher Andy Spielman and his colleagues had been studying the ecology of another tick-borne

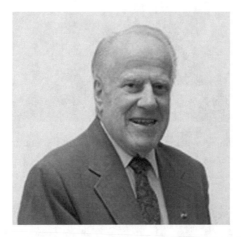

FIGURE 4. Willy Burgdorfer. *Source*: http://www.medicalecology.org/diseases/ lyme/lyme_disease.htm. Reprinted with permission.

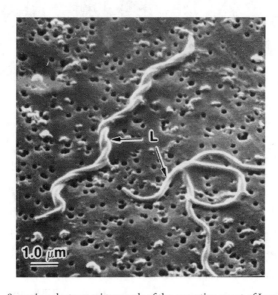

FIGURE 5. Scanning electron micrograph of the causative agent of Lyme disease, the spirochete bacterium *Borrelia burgdorferi*. *Source*: Wadsworth Center, New York State Dept of Health http://www.wadsworth.org/databank/borreli.htm. Reprinted with permission.

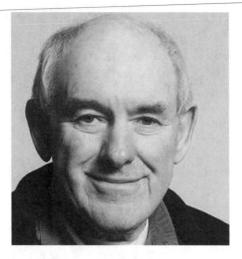

FIGURE 6. Andy Spielman. *Source*: Vector-Borne and Zoonotic Diseases (2007) 7:3. Reprinted with permission.

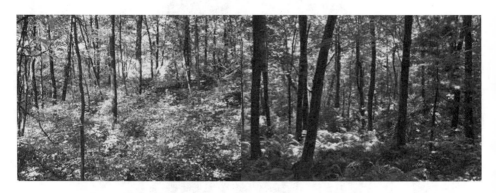

FIGURE 7. A typical forest understory that supports a high abundance of blacklegged ticks, the vector of Lyme disease in eastern and central North America. One hectare of this type of habitat in New England, the Mid-Atlantic, or the Upper Midwest might support hundreds to thousands of ticks.

zoonosis, human babesiosis, which occurred among residents of a few coastal New England communities (figure 6). Initially Spielman's group ascertained that *Babesia microti*, a protozoan parasite, was transmitted by *Ixodes scapularis* ticks that were common at their study sites on Nantucket Island and elsewhere (Spielman 1976). Later, Spielman and colleagues became convinced that the *Ixodes* species responsible for transmitting human babesiosis in coastal New England and New York was a previously unrecognized species distinct from *I. scapularis*, which they described and named *Ixodes dammini* (Spielman et al. 1979). This was ascertained to be the same species that in Long Island and elsewhere housed *B. burgdorferi* in its midgut, and it was abundant in forested and brushy habitats throughout southern New England and New York, including Lyme, Connecticut (figure 7). Tipped off by knowledgeable and persistent local residents and spurred by a strong public health concern, biomedical researchers had discovered what they thought was a new tick species and a new spirochete species, both of which were shockingly widespread and abundant.

The bacterial pathogen immediately suggested antibiotic therapy as the principal treatment for people already stricken with the disease. But for those not already ill, the importance of prevention and avoidance could not be overemphasized. Clearly, disease prevention would require knowledge of the biology of this "new" tick species. What was its life cycle? Where was it distributed? In what habitats and on what hosts could it be found? What regulated its abundance? By what means did ticks become infected with the spirochete? Pursuit of the answers to these questions would lead to the establishment of a simplified version of the ecology of the spirochetes, ticks, vertebrate hosts, and habitats involved in the maintenance and transmission of Lyme disease in North America. This simplified description has persisted tenaciously up to the present despite ample evidence that it is inadequate for understanding, predicting, or managing the dynamics of Lyme disease in humans and the natural environment. The following chapters describe the search for culprits on which to pin responsibility for the developing Lyme disease epidemic.

3

It's the Deer

MILLIONS OF PEOPLE IN NEW ENGLAND, NEW YORK, THE MID-Atlantic, and the Upper Midwest regions of the United States, not to mention many other localities in North America, Europe, and Asia, live in fear of contracting Lyme disease. They are aware that any time they picnic, hike, garden, walk the dog, or play catch they could encounter a tick and get seriously ill. The pervasive impression is that ticks are much more abundant than they used to be, that they are pretty much everywhere, and that deer are to blame because they are responsible for feeding the ticks and spreading them around. These notions are reinforced in virtually all accounts of Lyme disease and ticks provided by newspapers, television, and the Internet and are repeated in discussions with neighbors and friends. Deer are considered largely culpable for the sense of foreboding that can accompany each spring or summer foray from the house or apartment. The irritation at deer is only increased by their tendency to eat the flowers and shrubbery and dash out in front of cars. Many people are indignant that their towns or counties haven't done enough to manage deer and protect their health. In more and more of these towns, local people are organizing and pressuring governments to aggressively cull deer in order to reduce the Lyme disease threat.

Where did the notion that deer determine tick abundance and Lyme disease risk come from? What if it's wrong, or only partially right? What if culling deer—a very expensive and logistically challenging enterprise—does little or nothing to reduce risk of exposure to Lyme disease?

The notion that Lyme disease risk is closely tied to the abundance of deer arose from field studies that began shortly after the discoveries of the bacterial agent of Lyme disease and the involvement of ticks as vectors of these bacteria. The context of these studies was the hunt for the culprits— the *critical species*—involved in creating risk of exposure to Lyme disease. These were thorough and energetic studies, conducted with considerable urgency and scientific rigor. Such mission-oriented research can be a powerful weapon for fighting emerging infectious diseases, but the other side of this doubled-edged sword is the tendency to trim away complicating information before its importance can be evaluated. Perhaps it was the strong compulsion to provide specific information that could be used for disease prevention—in contrast to a quest for more basic information to support the understanding of general principles of disease risk and prevention—that led to this overly simplistic view of Lyme disease ecology.

White-tailed deer are considered "the definitive host of the [black-legged] tick" (Madhav et al. 2004), "the primary source of nourishment for gravid female *I. scapularis*" (Rand et al. 2004), "the primary reproductive stage host" (Rand et al. 2003), "the one indispensable piece in the LB [Lyme borreliosis] puzzle in North America" (Piesman 2002), and "the keystone host for adult *I. scapularis* (Childs 2009). In his excellent book on the history of Lyme disease medical research, Jonathan Edlow (2003: 149) makes note of the ancient existence of Lyme spirochetes and asks the question: "If the Lyme spirochete had been around for so long, why did it begin to surface as a recognized medical entity only in the past few decades? This question can be answered in one word—deer." Where did these conclusions come from, and what do they mean for Lyme disease ecology and prevention?

A flurry of research on what was then called *I. dammini* (see below) ensued in the late 1970s and 1980s to advance our understanding of risk factors for newly discovered Lyme disease and lay a foundation for preventive measures. Like other ixodid (hard) ticks, *I. dammini* was found to undergo two immature stages (larva and nymph) in addition to the adult stage (figure 8). At each stage, the tick takes a single blood meal from a vertebrate host to fuel transition to the next stage or, in the case of adults, to fuel reproduction. During these blood meals, the tick stays attached to the host's skin for several days to about a week, steadily imbibing host blood. Newly hatched larvae seek a host in midsummer, and after their blood meal, they drop off the host and molt into nymphs, which then overwinter on the forest floor before seeking a host the next late spring or early summer. After taking their blood meal, nymphs molt into adults,

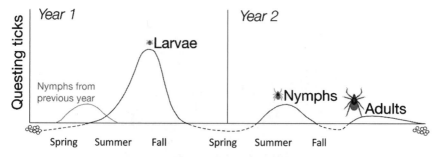

FIGURE 8. Basic life cycle of the blacklegged tick, *Ixodes scapularis*. This species was formerly and incorrectly called the "deer tick" (*Ixodes dammini*). Each year, a new cohort of larval ticks hatches from eggs in mid to late summer. After taking their single several-day-long blood meal from a vertebrate host, the larvae drop off, molt into nymphs, hunker down in the leaf litter or mineral soil, and overwinter on the forest floor. The next spring or early summer, these nymphs activate and seek a host (this is the stage mostly responsible for infecting humans and wildlife). After feeding on a host, the nymphs digest the blood meal, molt into the adult stage, and seek their final host in mid to late autumn. Thus, these ticks take three blood meals, once each as a larva, nymph, and adult, before reproducing and dying. *Source:* Brunner and Ostfeld (2008). Reprinted with permission.

which seek a host in mid to late autumn (figure 9). Adult females engorged with host blood overwinter before depositing an egg mass in spring, from which the next generation of larvae emerge in mid summer. When free-living on the forest floor (not attached to a host), these ticks are poor at getting about—they're able to crawl only a matter of meters. But they appear to be exquisitely sensitive to chemical and physical gradients, able to orient toward safe locations for overwintering and toward hosts emitting carbon dioxide and infrared radiation. Thus, the tick life cycle lasts two years and can involve three distinct vertebrate host species, with considerable time spent either inactive or seeking a host (*questing*) on the forest floor. The abundance and distribution of organisms with such complex life cycles could have been assumed to be determined by a complex suite of biotic and abiotic factors, including availability of several different hosts. However, even when first principles suggest that several factors are important in determining species abundances and how they change through time, such multifactorial approaches are rarely a part of initial research strategies (Lidicker 1991, Ostfeld 2008).

Several years before Lyme disease was recognized as a serious health threat, researchers began pursuing the ecology of another tick-transmitted disease that was attacking residents and visitors of Cape Cod and nearby islands such as Martha's Vineyard and Nantucket (Spielman

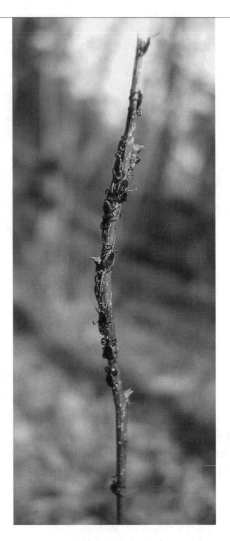

FIGURE 9. A group of adult blacklegged ticks in the act of *questing*—seeking a vertebrate host by climbing on forest-floor vegetation to a height of about 1 meter. As a potential host brushes against the vegetation, the ticks will grab hold of the animal and seek a site for attaching to the skin and drinking blood. Photograph by Michael Benjamin.

1976, Spielman et al. 1979) (figure 10). Medical entomologists working on Nantucket in 1976 and 1977 recruited Massachusetts Fisheries and Game Division personnel to shoot white-tailed deer year-round, and they also examined many deer shot by recreational hunters during the late autumn hunting season. Careful inspections of deer carcasses revealed large numbers of *Ixodes* ticks on various parts of the skin (Piesman et al. 1979). All three active life stages of the tick were abundant,

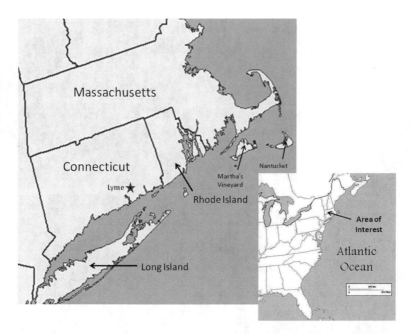

FIGURE 10. Map showing the coast of southern New England and adjacent New York, where Lyme disease first emerged in the 1970s. Cape Cod and the adjacent islands of Nantucket and Martha's Vineyard, the coast of Connecticut, and the north shore of Long Island were sites of particular importance as the seminal early studies of Lyme disease ecology got under way.

with larvae peaking in August (up to 467 per deer), nymphs peaking in June (up to 68 per deer), and adults most prevalent in November (up to 292 per deer). These researchers contrasted their results with those of the sparse prior literature on associations between ticks and their various hosts. This literature described immature *I. dammini* ticks as host specialists, being largely restricted to small rodents like mice and voles, and adult *I. dammini* as host generalists, being found on dogs, bears, foxes, skunks, opossums, raccoons, and other medium-sized and large mammals. Piesman and colleagues (1979) emphasized that their new findings suggested a very different scenario; the commonness of immature ticks on deer indicated that larval and nymphal abundances in fact might depend at least as much on deer as on small rodents, and the rarity of nondeer hosts on Nantucket indicated that adult ticks could be supported by deer alone (figure 11). This characterization of all tick life stages as closely tied to deer was highly influential and stimulated research on deer control as a method of reducing tick populations and the threat of tick-borne diseases.

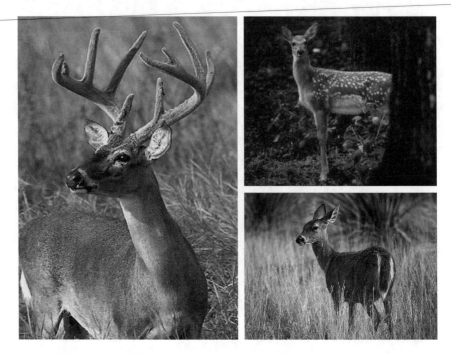

FIGURE 11. White-tailed deer, *Odocoileus virginianus. Source:* Myers et al. (2006). Reprinted with permission.

Strongly reinforcing this perception of deer as the critical host was the newly invented common (nonscientific) name "Dammin's northeastern deer ixodid"—later shortened to "deer tick"—applied to what was thought to be a newly described species, *Ixodes dammini* (Spielman et al. 1979). Initially, the tick species responsible for transmitting both Lyme disease and babesiosis in coastal New England was identified as *Ixodes scapularis*, the blacklegged tick (Spielman 1976, Wallis et al. 1978, Burgdorfer et al. 1982). This species was first described and named back in 1821 and had been found over the ensuing decades to be a very widespread tick species with populations documented from Massachusetts to Florida and from Ontario and Minnesota to Texas (Keirans et al. 1996) (figure 12).

For a species with such an enormous geographic range, some degree of variation in physical appearance among populations is to be expected, and indeed, considerable variation in morphological features thought to be tax-onomically important has been described (Oliver et al. 1993, Keirans et al. 1996). During the course of their Nantucket field studies of ticks and human babesiosis in the late 1970s, Spielman and colleagues (1979) became convinced that the northern populations of *I. scapularis* were sufficiently

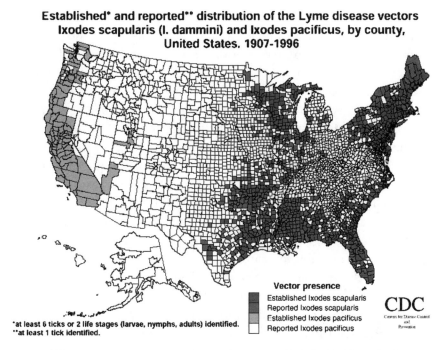

Established* and reported** distribution of the Lyme disease vectors Ixodes scapularis (I. dammini) and Ixodes pacificus, by county, United States, 1907-1996

Vector presence
- Established Ixodes scapularis
- Reported Ixodes scapularis
- Established Ixodes pacificus
- Reported Ixodes pacificus

CDC
Centers for Disease Control and Prevention

*at least 6 ticks or 2 life stages (larvae, nymphs, adults) identified.
**at least 1 tick identified.

FIGURE 12. Counties in the contiguousUnited States in which the blacklegged tick, *Ixodes scapularis,* has been collected. Also shown are the western counties where its close relative, the western blacklegged tick, *I. pacificus,* has been collected. *Source:* Dennis et al. (1998). Reprinted with permission.

distinct from southern populations to warrant the description of a new species, *I. dammini,* that was distributed from New England and New York to Ontario, Wisconsin, and Minnesota. This conclusion was based on differences between northern and southern populations in size, shape, and position of spines (auriculae) on the exoskeleton and in the apparent preference of immatures in northern populations for feeding on small rodents, in contrast to southern populations, which appeared to prefer lizards. Ultimately, neither the morphological nor the behavioral characteristics that were claimed to support the designation of a new species were justified.

Although the use of both morphological and behavioral characteristics to infer taxonomy has a rich history, these types of characteristics are also known to be unreliable in many instances. For example, differences between northern and southern tick populations in host associations could be caused by a variety of differences not related to taxonomy. Lizards are scarce and patchily distributed in some parts of these northern states and provinces and nonexistent in others; therefore, the ticks' lack of "preference" for lizards in these areas is not surprising. This leads to the question of how we ascertain which hosts ticks prefer to feed on. Rarely are ticks confronted with a choice between different host species that would allow their true preferences to be examined (but see Shaw et al. 2003). Instead, "preferences" are inferred from patterns of distribution of ticks on hosts. These patterns might be determined more by the relative availability of different host species in different areas than by innate preferences. (Interestingly, northern populations of these *Ixodes* ticks do in fact parasitize lizards where lizards occur [Giery and Ostfeld 2007].) Host associations also might be influenced by climate conditions that affect the specific locations where ticks dwell when seeking hosts. Surprisingly little research has been done on what preferences ticks might have for particular hosts and on what factors besides innate preferences affect the distribution of ticks on various host species that are available to them.

The conclusion that a new tick species had been discovered was rejected for a variety of reasons. Up until the 1970s, taxonomists relied primarily on morphological features to distinguish between related species. But taxonomists are fundamentally interested in separating species on the basis of their evolutionary, or *phylogenetic*, relationships, and morphological features can mislead scientists trying to infer these phylogenetic relationships. Many examples exist of organisms that cannot be distinguished morphologically, and so are lumped into the same species, that are later shown to consist of groups that are reproductively isolated from one another and therefore (by definition) distinct species. Similarly, many "species" are provisionally described on the basis of morphological differences from other related species but then are lumped into a single species when the groups are found not to be genetically distinct or reproductively isolated.

The dismantling of the status of *Ixodes dammini* as a distinct species began in 1993 with the publication of a comprehensive study by Oliver and colleagues (1993), who conducted laboratory mating experiments between "*I. dammini*" from Massachusetts and *I. scapularis* from Georgia. They found that these two species interbred readily and produced fertile offspring through at least three generations. In contrast, when either of these species was bred with another related *Ixodes* species—in this case *I. pacificus*—the mating resulted in hybrid sterility in the first generation. Oliver and colleagues also measured 65 different morphological characters in adults and nymphs of *I. dammini*, *I. scapularis*, and their "hybrid" offspring and found that statistical programs designed to discriminate between closely related taxonomic groups could not find distinguishing sets of characters and lumped the three groups together. Closely related species often differ in the size and arrangement of their chromosomes and in their versions of particular enzymes and proteins (isozymes), but neither chromosomes nor isozymes of the groups differed. Later comparisons of the DNA sequences for both ribosomes and chromosomes showed that *I. dammini* was not distinct from *I. scapularis* and that there was no evidence of reproductive isolation (Wesson et al. 1993, Norris et al. 1996). Norris et al. (1996) and Keirans et al. (1996) provide various lines of genetic and morphological evidence that all ticks previously thought to be *I. dammini* are actually *I. scapularis*, and that *I. scapularis* consists of two lineages, one that occurs from Florida to North Carolina (the "southern clade") and another that extends from Mississippi to New England (the "American clade"). The hypothesis that *Ixodes dammini* is a valid species has been discredited, and almost all scientists studying this species call it *Ixodes scapularis*. By the rules of zoological nomenclature, the common name "blacklegged tick" is the only correct vernacular name for this species.

But the 1979 description of the New England and New York ticks responsible for transmitting Lyme disease and human babesiosis as a new species, the deer tick *Ixodes dammini*, was accepted almost without dissention by tick biologists (*acarologists*), medical entomologists, epidemiologists, health care providers, and others. In the 14 years that elapsed before this taxonomy and associated names were invalidated, there was a veritable explosion of scientific research on these ticks, their hosts, and the pathogens they transmit. Much of the current understanding of the ecology and epidemiology of these diseases began during this period from the late 1970s to the early 1990s, when the tick was incorrectly named. Even today the invalidated common name "deer tick" persists in both the scientific and nonscientific literature. The persistence of this discredited name certainly helps perpetuate the notion that deer are the essential host for this tick.

The Science of the "Deer–Tick" Connection

Meanwhile, back in coastal New England in the 1980s, ticks were making many people ill, and scientists began to devise and evaluate means of controlling ticks. Given the pervasive view that deer were the critical host, these studies consisted of two basic approaches: (1) reducing, eliminating, or excluding deer from areas where ticks were abundant and disease risk high—an experimental approach; and (2) determining whether the abundance of ticks correlated with that of deer—a correlational approach. The first experimental reduction in deer density to assess impacts on ticks and disease risk was conducted by Mark Wilson and colleagues in 1982 on Great Island, Cape Cod, Massachusetts. They initially intended to capture deer, tranquilize them, apply insecticide/acaricide or tick repellents to their skin, and release them. These efforts proved both impractical and highly stressful to the deer, so instead this research group employed state biologists to shoot deer. Before removal, this 240-ha island supported an estimated population of at least 30 deer, and the experimental hunt reduced the deer population by an estimated 70%. To assess the impact of deer reduction on ticks, the researchers live-trapped white-footed mice (*Peromyscus leucopus*) and counted the larval and nymphal ticks on them. The results of Wilson and colleagues' study were disconcerting, to say the least. The dramatic reduction in deer abundance did nothing to decrease the number of ticks on mice, and there was even a suggestion that that number might be increasing (Wilson et al. 1984).

Later assessments of the impacts of deer reduction on tick abundance showed somewhat different results. Wilson and colleagues continued to reduce the deer population on Great Island throughout the mid-1980s until it was less than one-tenth of its previous size. At this point, the average number of larval and nymphal ticks on white-footed mice, and the total estimated population of immature ticks on the mouse population, declined significantly (Wilson et al. 1988). However, tick populations did not approach extinction on the island. On another coastal New England island, Monhegan Island in Maine, Rand and colleagues (2004) used hunters to remove deer, achieving their goal of complete eradication in the spring of 1999. By 2001, abundance of larval and nymphal ticks on Norway rats (*Rattus norvegicus*), the only apparent host for immature ticks on the island, declined to near zero, and by 2002 host-seeking adult ticks collected from vegetation became very scarce. On Long Island, New York, Duffy and colleagues (1994) surveyed tick abundance in 22 natural areas, seven of which had no deer. They found significantly fewer immature ticks in the deer-free sites, but all sites had nymphs, and the average number of nymphs collected in deer-free areas—10 per hour spent sampling—was within the range seen in areas with rampant Lyme disease.

Complete eradication of deer might be possible on some islands, but on the mainland it is infeasible, because deer-free zones are quickly recolonized by deer from neighboring areas. Consequently, researchers in mainland sites have sought to reduce rather than eliminate deer herds. On the Crane Reservation of coastal Massachusetts, Deblinger and colleagues (1993) used hunters to reduce the deer population from about 350 in 1985 to about 50 in 1991. Their counts of numbers of immature ticks on small mammals were initially encouraging, with larvae declining from about 21 per mouse before deer removal to about 10 per mouse after deer removal, and nymphs declining from about 3 to about 1.5 per mouse. But these reductions were only temporary, with numbers of both larvae and nymphs increasing in the early 1990s to levels similar to those measured before the deer reduction, despite the vastly reduced deer density at this time. On two sites in southern coastal Connecticut, Bridgeport and Bluff Point, Stafford and colleagues (2003) reduced deer density from more than 90 per square kilometer to about 15 to 30 per square kilometer. At Bridgeport, numbers of host-seeking nymphal ticks declined significantly after deer reduction, but numbers of host-seeking larvae fluctuated quite a bit, increasing in some years to near prehunt levels. At Bluff Point, the researchers found no significant correlation between abundance of host-seeking nymphs and abundance of deer, although abundance of larvae correlated with abundance of deer. At a suburban site in Somerset County, New Jersey, Jordan and colleagues (2007) assessed the impact of deer control by archery and shotgun hunters on tick populations. Hunters reduced the deer population by 47%, from about 46 to about 24 deer per square kilometer. However, abundances of both host-seeking larval and adult ticks at the culling sites were *greater* after deer reduction than before. Abundance of nymphs fluctuated with no apparent relation to deer culling. In addition, Jordan and colleagues assessed the impact of the deer reduction on numbers of Lyme disease cases reported to local health authorities and found no correlation between deer abundance and Lyme disease incidence in the township.

Logistically much easier and far less contentious than culling deer is excluding them from specified areas with deer-proof fencing. Several research groups have constructed deer exclosures to test the hypothesis that tick populations will be reduced where this host is excluded. The results of these studies have been striking in their inconsistency. In Westchester County, New York, one of two deer exclosures had a reduction in host-seeking nymphs compared to an unfenced reference site, whereas the other was not different from its reference site (Daniels and Fish 1995). In Lyme, Connecticut, deer exclosures reduced the abundance of host-seeking larvae and nymphs by more than 80% and about 50%, respectively (Stafford 1993). However, exclosures had no effect on abundance of host-seeking adult ticks, suggesting that the nymphs present in deer exclosures survived particularly well. In other cases, deer exclosures have strongly *increased* the abundance of host-seeking ticks of several species (including *I. scapularis*) compared to unfenced reference sites (Perkins et al. 2006). An intriguing synthesis of research on deer-exclosure impacts on ticks showed that small (~ 1-hectare) exclosures consistently *increase* tick abundances, whereas medium-sized exclosures (2–4 hectares) have no impact, and only those larger than about 4 hectares reduce tick populations (Perkins et al. 2006). These authors suggested that the exclusion of deer causes ticks that would have fed on deer to feed on other hosts, particularly small rodents. In small exclosures, these rodents can easily import ticks from the edges of surrounding unfenced areas into the interior of the exclosure, whereas in larger deer-free zones, tick importation declines in the interior (Perkins et al. 2006). It is also possible that exclusion of deer improves survival probabilities for ticks by protecting vegetation from intense browsing and increasing shading and moisture. It is critical to note that the threshold deer-exclosure size of 1–2 hectares, or 2–4 acres, within which tick populations are likely to increase corresponds closely to the size of individual private properties that people are likely to surround with fences in order to reduce Lyme disease risk.

Interestingly, whenever deer are eliminated, reduced by hunting, or excluded by fencing, the next several years sees an *increase* in the proportion of immature ticks that are infected with Lyme disease spirochetes (Rand et al. 2004, Perkins et al. 2006). Apparently, many of those immature ticks that would have fed on deer instead feed on other hosts, such as small mammals. Because deer are highly unlikely to transmit a spirochete infection to feeding ticks, but many small mammals are quite likely to transmit infection (more on this in chapter 4), the result is an increase in tick infection rates. Taking away deer, at least initially, removes the protective role they play in reducing tick infection (LoGiudice et al. 2003).

Even where deer populations have not been eliminated or reduced for experimental purposes, we know that deer populations naturally undergo ups and downs and vary from place to place, and one might expect that these changes might cause corresponding fluctuations in the tick population. On Long Island, New York, white-footed mice occupying forest sites that were used more intensively by deer were infested with more immature ticks than were those in sites used less intensively by deer (Wilson et al. 1990). Studies in coastal Maine showed that abundance of host-seeking adult ticks positively correlated with that of deer, and that these correlations occur both when many small sites are analyzed and when fewer, larger sites are examined (Rand et al. 2003). However, extensive, long-term studies in northern New Jersey (Schulze et al. 2001, Jordan and Schulze 2005) and southeastern New York (Ostfeld et al. 2006a) found no relationship between deer abundance and that of larval or nymphal ticks. In the latter case, deer abundance was estimated at six sites over a 13-year period.

Despite varying threefold among sites and years, deer abundance did not predict abundance of host-seeking nymphal ticks (Ostfeld et al. 2006a).

So, what do all these studies tell us about the relationship between deer and tick abundances? It is sometimes strong and sometimes weak or non-existent. It can vary from place to place. The different tick life stages respond inconsistently, as do host-seeking ticks and those attached to rodent hosts. The relationship might depend on the starting density of deer or of ticks. It seems to depend on the size of deer-free zones. It seems to be stronger in coastal or island localities than inland. Given the variable results described above, it is hard to support the conclusion that deer density and tick density are tightly coupled. The long-held, entrenched notion that deer are "indispensable," "primary," "keystone," and "definitive" needs to be replaced by a broader view of the factors responsible for regulating numbers of blacklegged ticks.

Why might the relationship between deer and tick abundance be so variable and sometimes weak or nonexistent? Ecologists expect species to be tightly coupled and their populations interdependent when one is a specialist on the other. For example, lynx are specialized predators on snowshoe hares; as hare populations go up, so too do lynx (after a time lag that corresponds to the lynx's generation time) (Elton 1966). But *Ixodes scapularis* is not a specialist on white-tailed deer. This tick species has been found on at least 125 species of North American vertebrates and is quite abundant on many of them (Keirans et al. 1996). Even the adult stage, which is frequently described as a specialist on deer, has been documented on 27 species of mammals (Keirans et al. 1996). Unfortunately, to my knowledge, no investigators have rigorously determined the relative abundance of adult blacklegged ticks on deer versus raccoons, opossums, skunks, foxes, and other common hosts on which they are regularly found. Ideally, such a study should be conducted by comparing among sites or among years in which deer abundance varies. When they seek a host, adult ticks climb understory vegetation to a height of roughly half a meter to a meter and grab hold of vertebrates that brush by (see figure 9). No one knows to what degree they are selective while questing—whether they avoid some hosts while favoring others or climb on the first host they encounter irrespective of species. If deer are the most abundant vertebrate in the size range that adult ticks encounter when questing, then more adult ticks might feed from deer than from other hosts. But if deer are scarce—whether from natural or anthropogenic causes—then more adult ticks might feed from these other nondeer hosts. Some of these hosts, such as opossums and raccoons, can reach abundances that exceed those of deer (see LoGiudice et al. 2003 and references therein). It seems reasonable to conclude that one reason tick populations are not always closely tied to deer populations is because the ticks have other hosts that can support them.

Deer that are killed by hunters in November are often infested with several dozen to more than a thousand adult blacklegged ticks (Main et al. 1981, Wilson et al. 1985). The female ticks embed their mouth parts and imbibe deer blood for up to a week, expanding from the size of a sesame seed to that of a small jellybean. During this time, the males wander over the deer, mating with the immobile females while sometimes taking brief blood meals to fuel their meanderings. Females that finish their blood meal drop off the deer and overwinter on the forest floor before laying a mass of about 2,000 eggs the next spring or summer. So a quick, back-of-the-envelope calculation shows that if a typical deer feeds a total of 2,000 adult ticks in any given autumn (500 per week for four weeks), of which one-half (1,000) are females, and half of all the eggs laid by those female hatch, the result from that one deer will be one million larvae. It quickly becomes evident that only a very small number of deer is necessary to produce astronomical numbers of ticks. If we double deer density, we get two million larvae; quadruple, and it's four million. But we don't find millions of ticks—of any life stage—in an area the size of a deer's home range. We might find up to a few thousand larvae in an area this size no matter how abundant deer are. Is it important whether the initial number of newly hatched larvae is four million or only one million, if a maximum of a few thousand will survive to seek a host? The point here is that other factors besides deer abundance are certainly involved in regulating abundance of ticks. Moreover, whatever these other regulatory factors are, they are likely to become increasingly important as the abundance of deer increases. This is simply because, if a relatively low threshold of deer abundance saturates the environment with ticks, then increasing density of deer above this threshold will not increase tick survival. Interestingly, the leading models of tick populations suggest that deer abundance thresholds *are* critical (Mount et al. 1997, Van Buskirk and Ostfeld 1995).

White-tailed deer have an enormous geographic range (Kays and Wilson 2002) that encompasses that of the blacklegged tick (figure 13). But deer were extirpated, or nearly so, over much of their range in the late 1800s to early 1900s as a result of rampant deforestation of the landscape and overhunting. Some deer survived, particularly in the southern United States, and deer populations elsewhere were reestablished by translocations (McShea et al. 1997). Over much of their eastern range, deer populations have increased in numbers and expanded during the twentieth century.

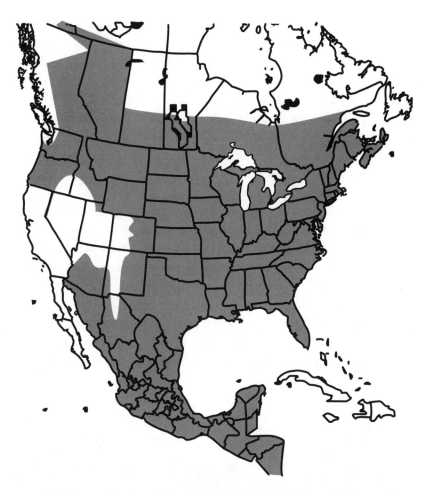

FIGURE 13. Geographic range of the white-tailed deer in North America. *Source:* Kays and Wilson (2002). Reprinted with permission.

When food is abundant, female deer can reproduce at two years of age and produce one or two fawns every year until they die. The ability of deer populations to grow quickly and expand in range has been attributed to regrowth of forests, combined with habitat fragmentation that created ideal habitat (juxtaposed forests and fields), plus the eradication of large predators such as cougars and wolves (McShea et al. 1997). It is dogma that the emergence of Lyme disease in the 1970s and 1980s was caused by the reestablishment of abundant deer populations after twentieth-century reforestation and predator decimation in the eastern United States (Spielman et al. 1985, Lane et al. 1991, Barbour and Fish 1993, among many others). The widely accepted scenario for the emergence of Lyme disease is that northern populations of blacklegged ticks survived in small refuges where the forest had never been completely cleared and thus deer had not been extirpated. The north shore of Long Island has been postulated as the main refuge (Barbour and Fish 1993, among many others). All around this refuge the forest regrew, deer habitat increased in quality, and deer reoccupied the landscape, setting the stage for ticks and Lyme disease to invade. Locations nearer to Long Island (for example, Lyme, Connecticut, which is just across Long Island Sound) were invaded earlier than those farther away.

Like many historical reconstructions, this scenario is probably impossible to evaluate rigorously. It seems plausible but also raises more questions than it answers. For example, deer and blacklegged ticks apparently survived the deforestation of the eighteenth and nineteenth centuries in many other locations in the southeastern, northeastern, south-central, and midwestern United States; why have these areas not seen similar invasions of Lyme disease? Why is there no correspondence at these large spatial scales between deer abundance and Lyme disease cases (figures 14 and 15)? Why was southern Connecticut invaded by Lyme disease in the 1970s, when deer had apparently been abundant for decades? More generally, why is there a long delay between the reestablishment of dense deer populations

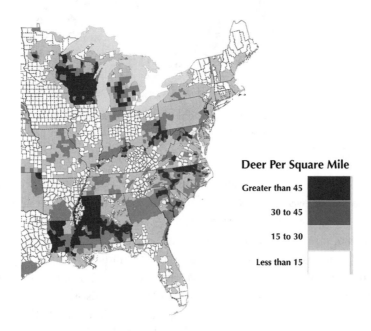

FIGURE 14. Distribution of deer population abundances in the United States. *Source:* The Quality Deer Management Association http://www.i-maps.com/Qdma/frame/ default1024_ie.asp?C=48449&LinkID=0&NID=0&cmd=map&TL=100000&GL=010100 &MF=11000. Reprinted with permission.

Annual Rate* of Lyme Disease by county of residence United States 1992 - 2006

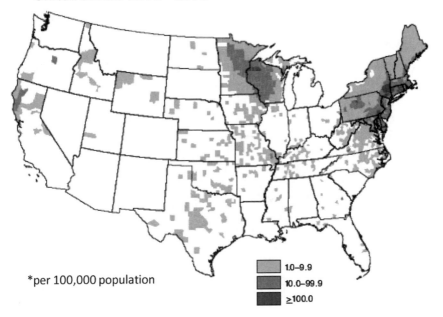

*per 100,000 population

	1.0–9.9
	10.0–99.9
	≥100.0

FIGURE 15. Distribution of Lyme disease incidence rates as reported to the United States Centers for Disease Control and Prevention by state health departments from 1996 to 2002. *Source:* CDC (2008). Reprinted with permission.

and that of Lyme disease, and why do these lag times appear to vary so dramatically from place to place? Perhaps, as discussed above, a particular threshold of deer density is necessary before tick populations and Lyme disease can be perpetuated, and the time lags reflect differences in when they exceed this threshold in different areas. But this notion does not by itself explain why ticks and Lyme disease don't occur in many areas with deer herds at least as abundant as in Lyme-endemic areas. Perhaps a threshold level of deer abundance is necessary but not sufficient; one also needs to have a massive influx of ticks—perhaps imported on migrating birds—to get the tick population off and running. But this by itself can't explain why Lyme disease is so rare in parts of the country with abundant deer and ticks. Perhaps it is necessary to have a threshold number of deer to support ticks, plus a source of tick importation, plus abundant wildlife species that feed the immature stages and are efficient at transmitting the Lyme disease spirochete to ticks (more about this in chapter 4). Notice that the scenario is getting increasingly removed from the notion that only one word—deer—is the answer to why Lyme disease has emerged when and where it has.

4

It's the Mice

IN SUMMER 1999 I RECEIVED A PHONE CALL FROM THE MAIN CARETAKER of the foxhounds, basset hounds, and beagles at the Millbrook (New York) Hunt Club, down the road from the Cary Institute of Ecosystem Studies where I work. This woman was distraught because her dogs were very sick—they were bleeding from their noses and mouths, losing their hair, having seizures, and wasting. She had contacted me because many of the sick dogs had tested positive for Lyme disease, for a disease then known as granulocytic ehrlichiosis (now known as granulocytic anaplasmosis), and for Rocky Mountain spotted fever. But distressingly, most of the hounds had not responded to antibiotics—a curious result given that all three of these diseases are caused by bacteria that are quite susceptible to standard veterinary antibiotics. Instead, more dogs were getting sick, and some were dying. The caretaker was contacting me—a field biologist—out of desperation, and there was essentially nothing I could do at the time.

Only after researchers from the U.S. Centers for Disease Control and Prevention and Walter Reed Army Institute of Research had tested various dog tissues for many pathogens was it discovered that the dogs were suffering from a disease called canine leishmaniasis (Gaskin et al. 2002), which is caused by a protozoan parasite called *Leishmania*. Various species of *Leishmania* cause terrible diseases in humans, as well as dogs, especially in South Asia, the Middle East, North and East Africa, and South America. *Leishmania* parasites are transmitted by tiny sand flies (*Phlebotomus* in the Old World and *Lutzomyia* in the New World). But given the tropical and subtropical distribution of these sand flies, it was quite strange that dogs as far north as Millbrook, New York, were suffering from canine leishmaniasis. One possibility was that a few dogs from the hunt club had been exposed to infected sand flies while on one of their road trips to the southeastern United States, where *Lutzomyia* sand flies are known to exist. (Foxhounds travel widely for hunting events.) Once the dogs had returned from their travels, these infected dogs perhaps had transmitted their parasites to their kennel-mates via saliva or other bodily fluids. Dogs in very close physical contact can transmit *Leishmania* parasites (Gaskin et al. 2002). Given the large number of dogs infected, though, this mode of transmission seemed improbable. The other main possibility was that sand flies and *Leishmania* do, in fact, exist in Millbrook, and the dogs were getting infected by these biting flies. Initial surveys conducted by sand fly experts at the site of the hunt club, however, revealed no sand flies (Ed Rowton, personal communication).

Adapting an old adage, I decided that the absence of evidence for sand flies was not the same as evidence for the absence of sand flies. So a group of disease ecologists, including Ed Rowton, Felicia Keesing, and I together with three interns, Lauren Canter, Wendy Haumaier, and Pamela Roy, decided that it would be worth a wider search for sand flies around Millbrook. In 2001 and 2002, these interns spent summer nights setting out fly traps that were baited with dry ice and a light source (figure 16). The dry ice emits carbon dioxide, which is a strong attractant for blood-feeding arthropods, and the light attracts various flying insects. Sure enough, we found *Lutzomyia vexator* sand flies (figure 17) at several of our locations on the campus of the Cary Institute, demonstrating that the Millbrook hounds might have been infected locally (Ostfeld et al. 2004). But what struck me, and the reason I have told this story, is that we also trapped thousands of *Anopheles quadrimaculatus* mosquitoes. This species' nontechnical name is the "common malaria mosquito," because it is a highly efficient vector of malaria parasites and was the main malaria-transmitting culprit in the United States until the 1950s, when malaria was wiped out in this part of the world. Yet, here it was in great abundance in Upstate New York in the twenty-first century. (The species is well known to occur throughout the eastern and central United States and even southern Canada, but this was news to me at the time.) Malaria is a very rare disease in the United States, and almost all cases diagnosed in this country were acquired by patients while they were traveling in tropical and subtropical places where malaria is endemic. The reason malaria is virtually never contracted within the United States is not because the vector is absent—it is resoundingly present—but because the *Plasmodium* parasite

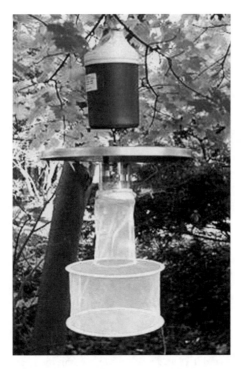

FIGURE 16. A "CDC light trap," baited with a light source and dry ice emitting carbon dioxide, both of which attract blood-feeding insects. A battery-powered fan sucks such insects into a collecting bag, which can then be retrieved the morning after deployment. These traps set at sites on the property of the Cary Institute of Ecosystem Studies in Millbrook, New York, captured abundant sand flies (*Lutzomyia vexator*) and common malaria mosquitoes (*Anopheles quadrimaculatus*), demonstrating the presence of competent vectors for serious human (and animal) diseases even where the disease might be scarce or absent. *Source*: http://www.ct.gov/mosquito/cwp/view.asp?a=3486&Q=414712&mosquito Nav=%7C. Reprinted with permission.

is absent. Clearly, in some cases the risk that humans will be exposed to a vector-borne disease is not reflected by the abundance of vectors that can transmit the parasite. Such risk might be better measured by the proportion of vectors carrying the parasite.

In the case of Lyme disease, the mere presence of the vector tick does not mean that risk of human exposure will be high, or even moderate. As shown in chapter 3, many parts of the eastern and central United States support abundant tick populations but experience very few cases of Lyme disease (see figures 12 and 15). One contributor to the rarity of Lyme disease in these areas is the low proportion of ticks that are infected with *Borrelia burgdorferi*. Understanding risk of Lyme disease requires that we

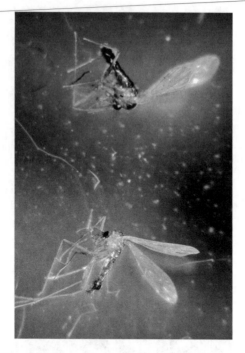

FIGURE 17. The sand fly, *Lutzomyia vexator*, a common inhabitant of the forests of Upstate New York. This species might have contributed to an outbreak of canine leishmaniasis and consequent illness and death of dozens of dogs. *Source*: Ostfeld et al. (2004). Reprinted with permission.

know not only what determines tick abundance but also what determines tick infection.

When *B. burgdorferi* spirochetes are present inside a blacklegged tick, they tend to remain in the intercellular spaces or attached to cell membranes along the lining of the midgut. Once the infected tick finds a vertebrate host and inserts its mouthparts into the host's skin, blood starts to flow into the tick's midgut. The presence of blood stimulates the bacteria to burrow through the lining of the tick's gut (apparently, the damage caused by this does not affect the tick's vitality) and enter the circulatory system, or *hemocoel* (pronounced "hee-mo-seal"). From the hemocoel the bacteria orient toward higher concentrations of blood, arriving at the tick's salivary glands within about 48 hours after the beginning of the blood meal. Once in the tick's saliva, the bacteria are injected into the host. So, it appears that in most cases *B. burgdorferi* is restricted to the tick's midgut, hemocoel, and salivary glands. However, in some samples of ticks, *B. burgdorferi* can spread to other tissues, including the reproductive organs. If able to infect tick ovaries, a pathogen has a second potential route outside the vector—it can exit when eggs are deposited by adult females. This is called *trans-ovarial transmission* and would result in newly hatched larval ticks being infected with the bacteria. However, both field-collected samples of larval *I. scapularis* ticks and larvae collected from mother ticks known to have fed on infected hosts are virtually never infected with *B. burgdorferi* (Piesman et al. 1986, Burgdorfer 1989, Sonenshine 1993, Patrican 1997). Evidently, in those cases when *B. burgdorferi* can invade tick ovaries, the spirochetes destroy the cells lining the oocytes, thus preventing shell formation and leading to the death of essentially all spirochete-infected eggs (Burgdorfer et al. 1989).

The fact that transovarial transmission of spirochetes from mother ticks to their offspring is rare to nonexistent means that ticks have essentially only one way of acquiring infection with *B. burgdorferi*. This sole mechanism is feeding on an infected vertebrate host. So, a critical question is: Which hosts are important in infecting ticks with the Lyme disease spirochete?

Even before the Lyme disease spirochete had been fully characterized and given a scientific name, researchers were seeking the identity of the host responsible for infecting ticks with this pathogen—that is, they were seeking the wildlife reservoir. The first such study assessed the ability of white-footed mice and white-tailed deer to act as *B. burgdorferi* reservoirs by Bosler and colleagues (1983). These researchers were aware that *Ixodes scapularis* ticks were reported from many species of mammalian hosts (Piesman and Spielman 1979, Carey et al. 1980), but they focused on these two hosts apparently because white-footed mice are ubiquitous and easy to capture from the wild, and because two fawns that had been killed by cars were readily obtainable for their studies. Bosler's group found spirochetes in the blood of both mice and deer. Furthermore, they found that 2 (8%) of the 25 ticks they collected from the fawns, and 113 (37%) of the 336 ticks they analyzed from the mice, were infected. They concluded that Lyme disease spirochetes were not host specific and that both deer and mice likely served as natural reservoirs. Follow-up studies a few years later showed that white-tailed deer are highly *inefficient* reservoirs, infecting on average only about 1% of the larval ticks that feed on them (Telford et al. 1988). In contrast, the focus zoomed in on white-footed mice, which were shown by several research groups to be highly efficient reservoirs (Anderson and Magnarelli 1984, Levine et al. 1985, Donahue et al. 1987).

White-footed mice are consistently shown to be the most efficient wildlife reservoirs of *B. burgdorferi*, infecting between 75% and 95% of larval blacklegged ticks that feed on them. However, several other host species are also competent reservoirs, including eastern chipmunks, short-tailed shrews, masked shrews, and American robins (Slajchert et al. 1997, Richter et al. 2000, LoGiudice et al. 2003, Brisson et al. 2008) (figure 18). All of these species can infect about 50% of feeding ticks, although the results of specific studies vary somewhat. One research group has suggested that some larger mammals such as raccoons are moderately efficient reservoirs (Fish and Daniels 1990), although other studies have found much lower transmissions rates for raccoons (Anderson and Magnarelli 1984, Mather et al. 1990, LoGiudice et al. 2003).

The mechanisms causing some vertebrate hosts to be more efficient than others at transmitting *B. burgdorferi* to feeding ticks are surprisingly poorly

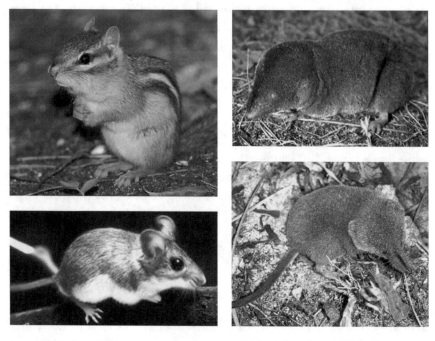

FIGURE 18. Some of the most competent reservoirs for *B. burgdorferi* within the range of the blacklegged tick. Clockwise from lower left are the white-footed mouse (*Peromyscus leucopus*), eastern chipmunk (*Tamias striatus*), short-tailed shrew (*Blarina brevicauda*), and masked shrew (*Sorex cinereus*). Sources: white-footed mouse (*Peromyscus leucopus*) http://animaldiversity.ummz.edu/site/resources/james_dowlinghealey/Mouse-house.jpg/view.html; eastern chipmunk (*Tamias striatus*) http://animaldiversity.ummz. umich.edu/site/resources/phil_myers/ADW_mammals/Rodentia/Tamias0005.jpg/view. html; short-tailed shrew (*Blarina brevicauda*) http://animaldiversity.ummz.umich.edu/ site/resources/phil_myers/classic/blarina_brevicauda.jpg/view.html; and masked shrew (*Sorex cinereus*) http://animaldiversity.ummz.umich.edu/site/resources/phil_myers/ classic/shrew3.jpg/view.html. Reprinted with permission.

understood. The probability that a given host will transmit the spirochetes to a feeding tick is a function of the abundance of spirochetes in the bloodstream (its *spirochetemia*). This in turn is a consequence of two main factors: whether the host has been exposed to infected ticks and, if exposed, the ability of *B. burgdorferi* to escape host immune defenses, proliferate, and persist. Within the major areas of endemic Lyme disease in the eastern and central United States, ground-dwelling forest mammals and birds are fed on by infected ticks at sufficiently high rates that virtually all such hosts are exposed to the Lyme spirochete. And indeed, even the least efficient reservoirs demonstrate that they are infected whenever they infect even a single feeding tick out of hundreds. (One important exception to this assertion is *co-feeding transmission*, which occurs when an infected tick feeds on the host in close physical proximity to an uninfected tick. In this situation, the pathogen can travel the short distance from infected to uninfected tick without proliferating and persisting in the host. Some pathogens, such as tick-borne encephalitis virus in Europe, appear to use this as the main means of transmission [Labuda et al. 1993].) So it appears that intrinsic, immunological differences among host species that regulate their spirochetemia are responsible for their varying efficiencies as reservoirs.

Western fence lizards, which abound in the California endemic zone for Lyme disease, are the quintessential *incompetent* reservoir for *B. burgdorferi* (Lane and Quistad 1998). These lizards use the complement pathway of their immune response to seek and destroy *B. burgdorferi* with circulating proteins that aggressively burst the bacterial cells. The complement proteins are ever-present (that is, they are part of the *innate* immune system rather than being induced after exposure to the pathogen) and are abundant enough that the first few microliters of blood imbibed by a feeding tick kill the spirochetes before they have a chance to leave the tick and enter the lizard host. However, the degree to which the complement system in other, nonlizard hosts is responsible for determining their efficiency as a spirochete reservoir is poorly understood. Recent research on European Lyme disease suggests that the ability of different species of mammal and bird hosts to maintain and transmit different species of *Borrelia* depends on whether their complement system tolerates that particular species (Gern 2008). But whether host-specific differences in the complement system are also responsible for different reservoir efficiencies for *B. burgdorferi* has not been established.

The other major immune pathway—that of *adaptive* immunity—is also involved in host responses to *B. burgdorferi*, but again, the specific mechanisms underlying species-specific differences in reservoir competence are not well understood (LaRocca and Benach 2008). For example, antibodies to *B. burgdorferi* are readily produced by all hosts within a few weeks after exposure and are detectable in blood samples taken from wild vertebrates and humans (Magnarelli et al. 1984). However, these naturally produced antibodies tend to be ineffective at clearing infections. Some antibodies, however, can be highly effective at clearing infections, as shown by the ability of vaccines against *B. burgdorferi* to prevent infection in humans and white-footed mice (Thanassi and Schoen 2000, Tsao et al. 2004). These vaccines consist of a purified protein found on the outer surface of *B. burgdorferi* cells called *outer surface protein A* (OspA). This antigen elicits the production of host antibodies that aggressively attack the spirochete. But hosts don't naturally experience OspA because the protein is produced by *B. burgdorferi* only when the bacteria are inside the tick, being down-regulated once the bacteria enter the host. Although the Lyme disease vaccine was specifically designed to elicit production of antibodies that are powerful killers of *B. burgdorferi*, some naturally occurring antibodies in wildlife hosts might also be effective. Species-specific variation in reservoir competence might depend on differences in antibody responses to infection, as well as on differences in the complement pathway.

A host that is a competent reservoir for *B. burgdorferi* will, by definition, cause infection in a high proportion of the ticks that feed on it in nature. However, if that host is rare, or if it is rarely bitten by ticks, then it might not contribute substantially to the total proportion of the tick population that is infected. This is because a high proportion of a tiny number is still a tiny number. To be a strong contributor to total tick infection prevalence, a host must also feed a substantial proportion of the tick population. Hosts that are abundant (many individuals per unit area) and that are heavily infested with ticks (many ticks per individual) will have the greatest impact on tick infection prevalence in nature. In fact, multiplying host population density by average tick burden per individual host will determine the total population density of ticks feeding on that host population (Giardina et al. 2000, LoGiudice et al. 2003). Multiplying this tick density by the host's reservoir competence (proportion of ticks feeding on that host that acquire infection) provides an estimate of the density of infected ticks produced by that host population (Mather 1993). If population density, average tick burden, and reservoir competence can be estimated for each of the host species fed upon by the tick population, then the proportion of ticks that feed on, and get infected from, each host species can also be estimated.

At the same time that the status of white-footed mice as Lyme disease reservoirs was being established, this species was also becoming implicated as the "primary," "principal," or "preferred" host for the immature stages of the tick vector (Piesman and Spielman 1979, Anderson and Magnarelli 1980, Main et al. 1982, Spielman et al. 1985). Individual mice caught in the summer are typically infested with 20 or 30 larval ticks at a time, sometimes many more (Brunner and Ostfeld 2008). And mice can be quite abundant in forest habitats, with numbers sometimes exceeding 50 per hectare (Ostfeld et al. 2006a). If a single host species is both the primary host for immature ticks and the principal reservoir for Lyme disease spirochetes, one might expect that species—the white-footed mouse—to be responsible for producing the great majority of infectious ticks (Mather et al. 1989). Indeed, Mather and colleagues (1989) concluded that white-footed mice were responsible for feeding more than 95% of the larvae that molted into infected nymphal ticks within their study sites in coastal Massachusetts. On the New England islands where most of the early descriptions of tick–host associations were conducted, few species other than white-footed mice are available for ticks to parasitize. Whether white-footed mice were also such a dominant species in other, more species-rich communities had not yet been established (Mather 1993). Nevertheless, as a result of these observations, it became axiomatic that the white-footed mouse is largely responsible for infecting blacklegged ticks with *B. burgdorferi* throughout the eastern North American Lyme disease zone (for example, Lane et al. 1991, Piesman 2002).

Curiously, counts of immature ticks on white-tailed deer, eastern chipmunks, squirrels, opossums, raccoons, skunks, foxes, and other hosts were sometimes shown to exceed those on white-footed mice (Anderson and Magnarelli 1984, Fish and Daniels 1990, Telford et al. 1990). But the importance of these hosts in producing infected ticks had been largely discounted because the tick burdens on these hosts seemed inadequate to compensate for the hosts' relatively low population densities. And in addition to the relatively low total density of ticks expected to be fed by these species, all of them were known to have low transmission efficiencies of *B. burgdorferi* to ticks, compared to mice.

My research group has set and checked many hundreds of thousands of live animal traps over the years (figure 19). When we catch a white-footed mouse, we remove the animal from the trap and hold it by the scruff of the neck to check its sex, breeding condition, identity (the number on its ear tag), body mass, and the number of ticks that are attached to it. For some unknown reason, blacklegged ticks on mice

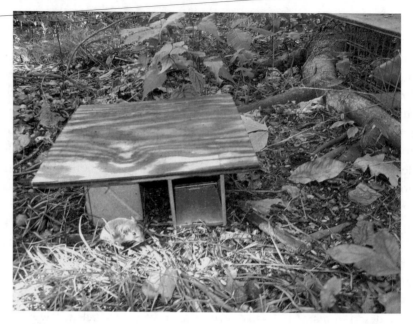

FIGURE 19. Sherman live traps set on the forest floor at study sites in Millbrook, New York. The metal traps are baited with oats and covered with a board for protection. They are baited in the evening and checked early the next morning. Animals in the traps are marked with a numbered ear tag, inspected for sex, age, breeding condition, tick burdens, and body mass, and then released at the site of capture. Note the white-footed mouse with an ear tag in front of the closed trap on the left.

orient toward the ears, which are big and only sparsely covered with fur (figure 20). By carefully inspecting the ears and face of a mouse for about one minute, we detect about 90% of the ticks that are attached to it. We know this because we have retrieved hundreds of mice to the lab and held them in wire mesh cages (supplied with water and their favorite foods) over pans of water for up to 5 days, longer than larval blacklegged ticks typically stay attached before they drop off the host. (The pans of water beneath cages contained much more than just ticks—this was a messy and challenging task, but sometimes we must make sacrifices for science.) So we have a full count of tick burdens on many individual mice that we also inspected in the field. Repeating the same process for chipmunks (*Tamias striatus*), we know we detect about 60% to 75% of the ticks during our one-minute inspections in the field. For all other mammal and bird hosts we trap, counts in the field are such wild underestimates that we don't even bother. Blacklegged ticks on these other hosts tend to distribute themselves over the entire body, where fur or feathers can be

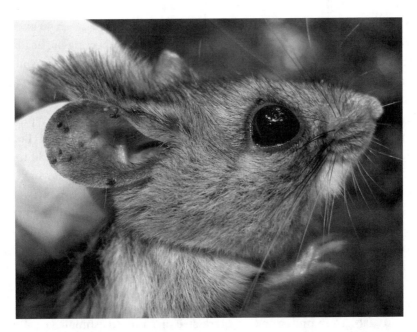

FIGURE 20. A typical white-footed mouse as captured in midsummer. Its ears
are covered with larval blacklegged ticks. Direct counts of ticks on the ears and
face of mice are highly efficient, typically identifying about 90% of the total
number of ticks on the whole body. For unknown reasons, the same is not
true of other hosts, for which direct counts in the field are gross underestimates
of total body burden. Photo by Jesse Brunner.

dense and thick and the ticks are impossible to see. If hosts are anesthetized,
they can be inspected somewhat more carefully, but even these counts tend
to grossly underestimate actual tick burdens (Fish and Daniels 1990).

Unaware of the inaccuracies, many of the influential early studies enu-
merating tick burdens on various vertebrate hosts conducted direct counts
of field-caught individuals (Piesman and Spielman 1979, Carey et al. 1980,
Main et al. 1981, Anderson et al. 1983, Fish and Dowler 1989, Telford et al.
1990). These studies tended to conclude that white-footed mice were the
principal or preferred host of immature (especially larval) ticks without
being aware of the wide differences in probabilities of detecting ticks on
different hosts. A critical observation was published by Fish and Daniels
(1990), who found that only 11% of the larvae on raccoons and 13% of
those on skunks were detected during careful inspections of anesthetized
animals. And these values are surely quite conservative—their estimate of
the "true" tick burden on mammalian hosts was based on the number
counted in pans of water beneath cages after holding the animals for only
24 to 48 hours in the laboratory. Our studies (Keesing et al. 2009) show

that as many as 50% of the ticks on a host can drop off between 48 and 72 hours after the host is captured. Similarly, based on inspecting the heads of field-caught short-tailed shrews, Telford and colleagues (1990) concluded that this species was rarely infested with blacklegged ticks, and those that were infested had very low burdens. However, my research group has found that visual inspections of live or recently deceased shrews typically underestimate actual tick burdens by about an order of magnitude (LoGiudice et al. 2003, Brisson et al. 2008). It is not unusual to collect 30 to 50 larval ticks in a pan held beneath a captive field-caught shrew on which we counted only a handful during close examination in the field. The overall result of these biases is that, during the first decade or two after the Lyme disease spirochete and vector were discovered in New England and New York, most of the published data concerning tick burdens on nonmouse hosts probably were moderate to gross underestimates. But the same was not true of tick-burden estimates on white-footed mice, which tended to be more accurate.

My lab group undertook an aggressive program to estimate larval tick burdens on as many vertebrate hosts as possible inside an intensely endemic zone for Lyme disease. This program was led by Kathleen LoGiudice, who ran herself ragged for several summers in the forest setting traps and nets of all sizes and retrieving mammals and birds to the lab to collect ticks from pans of water held beneath cages. With the exception of ground-dwelling birds (veery, wood thrush, gray catbird, American robin), we found that each of the host species we captured had more larval ticks per individual than did mice (figure 21). Even the tiny masked shrews (*Sorex cinereus*) (~5 grams, averaging 55 ticks) had about twice as many ticks per individual as did mice (~20 grams, 28 ticks). Of course, knowing the average number of larval ticks on a particular host species is insufficient for projecting how important that host is in feeding the tick population. For example, we found about 70 ticks on the average skunk, but we also estimated that there is about one skunk per 20 hectares of forest, so skunks are not contributing huge numbers of ticks to the forest floor. On the other hand, the average short-tailed shrew hosts about 63 larval ticks, and we estimate about 25 shrews per hectare of forest. These data allowed us to apportion larval tick meals and nymph infection events among the various host species that we were able to capture (LoGiudice et al. 2003; more on this below). Complicating our attempts to estimate the number of larval ticks fed, and nymphal ticks produced, by each species of host is the uncomfortable fact that some of these species fluctuate in abundance quite dramatically from year to year. These population fluctuations are most

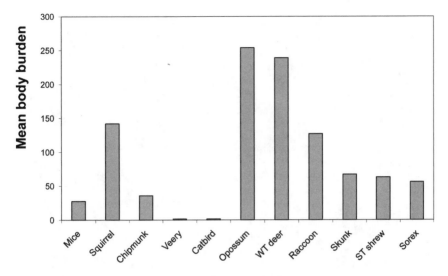

FIGURE 21. Average numbers of larval blacklegged ticks (body burdens) found on mammals and birds captured in a Lyme-disease-endemic area in Millbrook, New York, in mid to late summer. WT deer = white-tailed deer; ST shrew = short-tailed shrew. *Source*: Updated from LoGiudice et al. (2003).

pronounced for the small mammals like mice, chipmunks, and probably shrews.

But the upside of having host populations that naturally fluctuate is that one can ask whether changes in abundance of particular hosts cause changes in the abundances or infection rates in ticks without having to experimentally manipulate the system. Heavily influenced by the field and laboratory studies from the 1980s showing the high reservoir competence and tick burdens of white-footed mice, I established a study in 1991 to ask whether fluctuating mouse populations caused fluctuations in numbers of infected ticks. We started with two large (2.25-hectare) trapping grids on the grounds of the Cary Institute of Ecosystem Studies and later phased in four more grids. Approximately monthly between May and November of each year, we captured, marked, and released any small mammal that entered our live traps and gathered standard data that allowed us to esti-mate population size, tick burdens, and individual traits. The species we trapped most commonly were white-footed mice, eastern chipmunks, and short-tailed shrews, although we occasionally captured weasels, sparrows, baby opossums, voles, flying squirrels, and even young mink. To monitor tick populations, we started by sampling the forest floor every few weeks from April to November to determine the host-seeking activity periods for larvae, nymphs, and adults (figure 22). Similar to other nearby sites (Fish

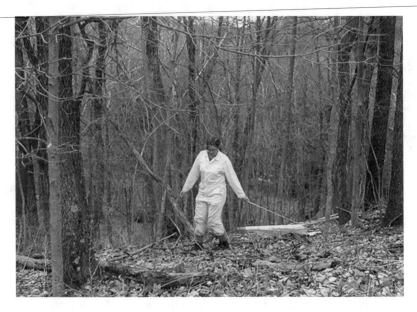

FIGURE 22. A research technician sampling the forest floor and understory for ticks using a drag cloth. Drag cloths consist of 1-square-meter pieces of white corduroy cloth with weights sown into the far end and a wooden dowel holding the near end flat. Researchers pull a tow rope attached to the dowel along premeasured routes and count ticks at regular intervals. Ticks readily attach to the cloth as it brushes by, mimicking a vertebrate host as it moves along the forest floor.

1993), we found that activities of nymphs peaked in mid to late June, larvae in mid August, and adults in late October to early November. Once this seasonality was established, we focused our sampling at those activity peaks. To count ticks, we use a low-tech but reliable method called drag sampling. We use one-square-meter pieces of white corduroy cloth with a wooden dowel sewn along one side and steel weights sewn into the opposite side. A tow rope attached to the dowel side allows it to be pulled slowly along premeasured routes, and the weights keep the cloth pressed against the ground or understory vegetation. Because we are interested in understanding variation in human risk of exposure to Lyme disease, we focus on nymphs (which are responsible for the vast majority of Lyme disease cases; Barbour and Fish 1993, many others). In addition to counting the ticks, we subject nymphs and adults to assays to determine what proportion of them are infected with *Borrelia burgdorferi*.

When we started this monitoring, we predicted that the proportion of nymphs infected with *B. burgdorferi*, or what we call *nymphal infection prevalence* (NIP), each year would strongly correlate with the abundance of white-footed mice the prior year. Because white-footed mice are the most competent reservoir for the Lyme disease spirochete, we expected that when mice were abundant, a high proportion of the larval ticks would be able to feed on mice, leading to a high proportion of those ticks becoming infected. The lag time of one year was expected because these larvae become active as nymphs about one year later. If mice are also a superior host for larval ticks, in the sense that larvae feeding on mice have a higher probability of surviving than do larvae feeding on other hosts, then we might also expect that the *density of nymphs* (DON) would be higher one year after a good mouse year. If both NIP and DON correlate with last year's mouse abundance, then the *density of infected nymphs* (DIN) should be predictable from last year's mouse population. All three of these parameters, NIP, DON, and DIN, are predictors of human risk.

After 13 years of monitoring, we were surprised to find that, although NIP seemed to positively correlate with mouse abundance in the prior year, this relationship was weak and not statistically significant (Ostfeld et al. 2006a). This same weak relationship held when we added chipmunks—the second most competent reservoir—to our statistical models. Instead, mouse abundance was a significant predictor of both DON and DIN, suggesting that mice are a particularly high-quality host for larval ticks. But our statistical models showed two unexpected results: that mouse abundance explained only about 58% of the variation in DON and DIN, leaving quite a bit of the variation unexplained, and that chipmunk abundance was as good a predictor of DON and DIN as was mouse abundance (Ostfeld et al. 2006a) (figure 23). (Several years later our group demonstrated that larval ticks survive best when they feed on mice and second best when they feed on chipmunks, with most other hosts managing to kill most ticks by grooming them off when the ticks attempt to feed [Keesing et al. 2009].) The importance of chipmunks surprised us because they are only about half as abundant as mice are each year, and they are not as efficient a reservoir as mice are. Yet our concurrent studies (LoGiudice et al. 2003, Ostfeld and LoGiudice 2003) showed that they feed more larval ticks on average than mice do.

Both mice and chipmunks are attracted to the live traps we set on the forest floor. The traps are boxlike, sheet-metal contraptions provided with oats as bait and a plywood cover board for shading and rain protection. Many small rodents like mice and chipmunks are drawn to dark holes, especially if they smell of food and other critters (we leave the traps in place year-round, so they accumulate rodent scent). Because we have good estimates of how many mice and chipmunks dwell within our trapping grids

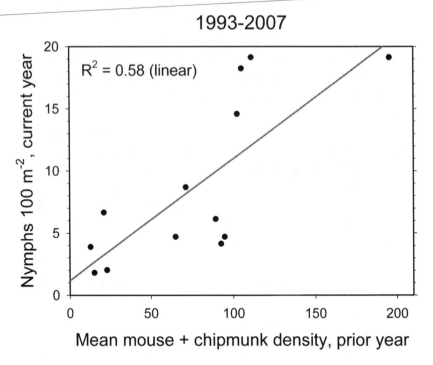

FIGURE 23. The relationship between the combined abundances of white-footed mice and eastern chipmunks from each year and the density of nymphal ticks (DON) the next year. Data are from long-term monitoring of mammal host and tick abundances on six large (2.25-hectare) field plots at the Cary Institute of Ecosystem Studies in Millbrook, New York. DON strongly correlates with abundances of these rodents the previous summer.

at any given time, we can estimate what percentage of them get caught during any given weekly trapping session. For mice this is around 90%, and for chipmunks it is 60% to 70%. Unfortunately, for some other common small mammals, these traps are not terribly attractive, and we suspect (but can't confirm) that we catch only a small fraction of the animals alive on the grid at any given time. Short-tailed shrews and masked shrews will occasionally walk into a trap and spring it shut, allowing us to gather data on tick burdens and reservoir competence, but we have little confidence that capture numbers reflect actual numbers. Estimating their abundances is made even harder by the absence of external ears in short-tailed shrews, which prevents our use of individually numbered ear tags. So estimates of shrew population abundance need to be viewed with caution. Shrews that we do capture are quite challenging to keep alive in the laboratory, because their extraordinarily high metabolic rates mean that they need massive quantities of food (usually dozens of mealworms) and water (saturated bits of sponge work best) each day. I strongly suspect that these logistical challenges pertaining to shrew trapping and husbandry, as opposed to actual data, are responsible for the commonly held belief that these hosts are relatively unimportant in Lyme disease ecology.

Nevertheless, given that we have estimates of average tick burdens, population densities, and reservoir competencies of most of the important mammal and bird hosts at a typical Lyme disease site, we can calculate the proportion of all larval meals, and of infected nymphs, that are contributed by each species, including shrews. We are confident in our estimates of average tick burdens and reservoir competence of short-tailed shrews and masked shrews, but much less so in estimates of their average population densities. With these uncertainties in mind, our calculations (based on the data in LoGiudice et al. 2003, 2008) suggest that short-tailed shrews and masked shrews, together, feed about 40% of all the larval ticks that find a host. Perhaps even more surprising is our estimate that the two shrew species are responsible for more than half of all the infected nymphs in the environment. The same data set indicated that white-footed mice were feeding only about 15% of larval ticks and infecting less than 20% of the larvae that become infected nymphs. If we are overestimating shrew abundance, then our estimates of these percentages for shrews will decline and those for mice might increase.

A critical follow-up study to trace the source of larval tick blood meals and nymphal tick infections was led by Dustin Brisson. Brisson and colleagues, together with other research groups, discovered that the species *Borrelia burgdorferi* (*sensu stricto*; that is, excluding related species of *Borrelia* that are sometimes lumped with *B. burgdorferi* but that do not cause Lyme disease) consists of 22 different strains, or genotypes, of which 15 occur in the northeastern United States endemic zone for Lyme disease. These genotypes are identified based on differences in one location, or *locus*, in the bacterium's genome, called *ospC* because it codes for outer surface protein C (OspC). This locus is at least 10 times more variable than any other genetic locus in *B. burgdorferi*, so it provides information on how this bacterial species has split into distinct genetic and evolutionary units. *Borrelia burgdorferi* begin to turn on the *ospC* genes and produce OspC protein while they are in the tick, shortly after the tick begins to feed on a vertebrate host. OspC continues to be produced while *B. burgdorferi* migrates from the tick's midgut to its salivary glands and finally into the vertebrate host (see Brisson and Dykhuizen 2004 and references therein). Consequently, it is one of the first antigens detected by the host immune system and becomes the target of antibody production. For reasons that are poorly understood, the different species of vertebrate hosts vary in their ability to attack and destroy *B. burgdorferi* carrying different *ospC* genotypes. Each host can clear initial invasions by most *B. burgdorferi* genotypes but permits invasion by the others, and the set of genotypes that can invade is different for white-footed mice versus chipmunks, short-tailed shrews, masked shrews, gray squirrels, and other hosts. These differences among hosts are not absolute, however. For example, the genotypes that can persist in mice include *ospC* types A, B, D, F, G, I, and K, whereas chipmunks support *ospC* types A, D, F, G, I, K, T, and U (Brisson and Dykhuizen 2004). Despite the presence of *B. burgdorferi* strains that persist in more than one host species, each of the five well-characterized mammal hosts supports a unique constellation of genotypes.

Brisson and colleagues (2008) started by characterizing the genotype frequencies present in hundreds of host-seeking nymphal ticks from sites in Dutchess County, New York. These host-seeking nymphs are responsible for inoculating all of the vertebrate host species (including humans), so one expects that each host will be exposed to each *B. burgdorferi* genotype in proportion to its frequency in the questing nymph population. Brisson's group then collected larval ticks from pans held beneath cages of mice, chipmunks, squirrels, short-tailed shrews, and masked shrews, allowed those larvae to molt into nymphs, and determined which *B. burgdorferi* strains were present. Data for each species on what strains they were exposed to (from questing nymphs), and what strains they transmitted to feeding larvae, allowed the calculation of transmission probabilities for each strain by each host. With these data in hand, Brisson and colleagues then went out and collected a new batch of questing nymphs from the forest floor and used statistical methods to assign each nymph to a particular host species. Because larval ticks are not born with a *B. burgdorferi* infection, each questing nymph must have obtained its particular constellation of *B. burgdorferi* genotypes from the blood meal it took as a larva. Each nymph's constellation of *B. burgdorferi* genotypes could be assigned to a particular host species with a particular probability, given the transmission probabilities that had been calculated for the individual strains.

This combination of molecular and ecological data and statistical modeling strongly supported the hypothesis that shrews are far more important in feeding and infecting immature ticks than had been realized. Brisson and colleagues (Brisson et al. 2008) found that the two species of shrews together hosted about 30% of all the larval ticks that fed successfully, and these shrews infected about 55% of the larvae that molted into infected nymphs. On the other hand, white-footed mice fed 10% to 15% of larval ticks, with this number increasing in high-mouse-density years, and infected between 25% and 30% of the population of infected nymphs. Chipmunks feed between 6% and 10% of all larvae and provided between 10% and 15% of all infected nymphs. Altogether, 80% to 90% of all the infected nymphs at this typical Lyme disease site took their larval blood meal from a mouse, a chipmunk, a short-tailed shrew, or a masked shrew (figure 24). However, these four host species together fed fewer than half of the total larvae that survived to the nymph stage.

Given these results, it is perhaps not surprising that yearly variation in the abundance of mice and chipmunks explains only about half of the yearly variation in the density of infected nymphs on the forest floor. If we were able to accurately monitor shrew populations, I suspect that we'd be

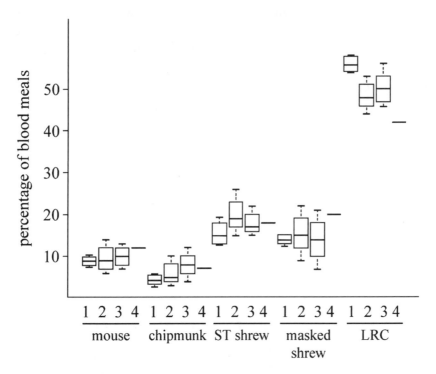

FIGURE 24. Estimated percentage of blood meals taken from white-footed mice, eastern chipmunks, short-tailed shrews, masked shrews, and the remainder of the host community, termed *LRC* for low-reservoir-competence hosts. Each horizontal line and surrounding bar represent the average and standard deviation, respectively, of an independent estimate based on molecular or ecological data. Note the similarity between estimates from different methods of estimation (for details, see Brisson et al. 2008). *Source*: Brisson et al. (2008). Reprinted with permission.

able to explain considerably more of this variation. Nevertheless, we are left with several important conclusions. One is that the assertion that white-footed mice are the principal, primary, or preferred host for immature blacklegged ticks and principal reservoir for *B. burgdorferi* cannot be supported. Inconspicuous hosts can sometimes be at least as important as the usual suspects, such as white-footed mice, that are the easiest to catch and inspect for ticks. A related conclusion is that predicting how many infected nymphs will occur in any given time and place might require knowledge of the entire community of hosts rather than of only one or two species. While our group of four species of rodents and shrews is feeding nearly half of all the larvae in the forest, and infecting about 90% of the ones that get infected, all the other hosts are feeding more than half of the larvae and infecting only 10% of them. Each larval tick that doesn't get infected because it feeds on one of these reservoir-incompetent hosts— raccoons, skunks, opossums, deer, squirrels, veeries, wood thrushes, and so on—will molt into a nymph that will not transmit *B. burgdorferi* to another host, including humans. Perhaps the southern and midwestern portions of the United States, which have widespread blacklegged tick populations but few Lyme disease cases, are under the protection of abundant nonrodent, nonshrew hosts. We'll return to this theme in chapter 8.

5

It's the Weather

IMAGINE THAT YOU'RE AN INTELLIGENT BEING FROM A DISTANT PLANET on a reconnaissance mission to Earth in the late seventeenth century, local time. You park your spacecraft just outside Earth's atmosphere above eastern North America and train your remote sensing equipment on the land below. You're aware from previous missions that a group of *Homo sapiens* has recently invaded from across the great ocean to the east. This group of transoceanic dispersers is somewhat mobile and shows the potential to invade elsewhere on the continent. They're a rather bloodthirsty lot and have already done substantial damage to some of the native North American flora and fauna, including the native *H. sapiens*, and this causes concern to your species. Your mission is to estimate how far into the new continent they will disperse and permanently settle. They appear to suffer from disease and high mortality during the very cold and very hot times of year, and whenever there are long periods of flooding or drought. So you deduce that the major constraint on their distribution is the climate.

You notice that this group of *H. sapiens* seems to be largely limited to the zone within a few hundred kilometers of the east coast, and you create a detailed map of this distribution. Your map superimposes a line on the continent within which the group occurs and outside of which it doesn't. Using the remote sensing equipment onboard your spacecraft, you measure seasonal temperature and precipitation minima, maxima, and averages inside and outside the occupied zone. Using statistical algorithms, you determine the combination of temperature and precipitation variables that best describes the mapped area that this group currently occupies.

You statistically evaluate different combinations of variables and don't stop until you arrive at one with very high explanatory power. You confirm this by determining that your combination of variables almost never occurs where the *H. sapiens* are absent (high *specificity*), and that places with that combination almost always have *H. sapiens* populations (high *sensitivity*). Because they occupy only this part of the continent, you presume that this particular combination of temperature and precipitation variables is conducive to their survival and other combinations are not.

Next, you entrain your remote sensing equipment on the rest of the continent. Your purpose is to determine where else the climatic conditions will allow this group to settle. You find large zones in the middle portions of the continent that match your variables and are suitable, but even more extensive areas farther west that don't match and are unsuitable. So, you project that, if the group of *H. sapiens* is able to get there using their rudimentary transportation modes, it will move in a broad wave westward a thousand kilometers or so where the climate is still suitable, but not beyond. The native flora and fauna of the western, southern, and northern parts of the continent will therefore be safe from this destructive population. You return to your planet to spread news of your findings.

Two hundred years later you return to Earth to check on how far these *H. sapiens* have moved. You're shocked to find that they occupy pretty much the entire continent; you grossly underestimated how far west, south, and north they would be able to settle. Their impact has been tragic. Where did you go wrong? In order to find out, you must infiltrate this population and understand how they are able to live in areas you were quite certain were entirely inhospitable. You soon determine that you made three assumptions that turned out to be unfounded. First, you had assumed that climatic variables were the only important determinants of the population's geographic range and that interactions with other species (*biotic* interactions) were unimportant. But close study revealed that this species is intimately connected with other organisms such as cows, chickens, and wheat plants, which they were able to bring with them as they dispersed, expanding the hospitable range. Second, you assumed that the genotypes and phenotypes of the population were fixed and would not change as it expanded its range. But your later study revealed that the population changed its diet (for example, ate more fat in northern climes), its daily activity patterns (took midday naps in more southern and western climes), its site selection for dwellings (placed in clearings in forested biomes and surrounded with trees in nonforested biomes), and its external coverings (thicker in the north, thinner in the south and west). These phenotypic changes allowed the population to adapt to, or avoid, challenging physical conditions. Third, you assumed that the group occurred in all locations where the climate was favorable and nowhere else. Your later research showed, however, that the *H. sapiens* population in the late seventeenth century occupied only a small subset of the climates that were favorable, because it had arrived on the continent only recently and had limited powers of dispersal. Therefore, the map you so painstakingly prepared and statistically validated encompassed only a subset of the climates suitable for the population, and your continent-wide projections were gross underestimates.

This basic methodology used by our intergalactic visitor is commonly used here on Earth by scientists interested in predicting where species will likely expand their geographic ranges. Species that are strong candidates for analyses like this are nonnative species that are invading new areas, those that are reinvading areas from which they were eliminated or strongly reduced, and those that appear sensitive to the rapidly changing climatic conditions caused by greenhouse gas emissions. Blacklegged ticks in North America would seem to fall into the latter two categories.

Around the time of the discovery of Lyme disease, it was thought that blacklegged ticks were restricted to low-elevation coastal sites in New York and New England because fall and winter temperatures at locations higher in elevation and farther inland prohibited their survival (McEnroe 1977). The discovery of healthy populations of blacklegged ticks in considerably colder climates of Minnesota and Wisconsin, combined with the spread of coastal New England populations into the interior, soon discredited this notion. The realization that blacklegged ticks and Lyme disease could exist under a much broader range of climatic conditions than suggested by their current distribution was critical but underappreciated by many later research efforts. If the current range of the tick is only a fraction of its potential range, then the climatic variables inside its current range represent only a subset of the range of conditions that can support tick populations. In other words, any snapshot of a species' distribution, when that species is in the process of expanding, says little or nothing about the range of conditions in its eventual geographic range. But projections based on such snapshots have been commonplace in the intervening years.

In a pioneering early study of the potential climatic factors limiting the distribution of blacklegged ticks, Estrada-Peña (1998) used remote sensing images from NOAA satellites to characterize climatic conditions throughout North America thought to be important to blacklegged ticks. The variables selected were ground-level temperature minima and maxima and a common index, the *normalized difference vegetation index*, or NDVI, throughout North America. NDVI represents "greenness" of the vegetation and therefore integrates seasonal temperature, precipitation, soil type, vegetation type, and other variables. Of course, temperature conditions and NDVI vary seasonally, so the data were divided into 10-day intervals covering the entire year. Estrada-Peña then placed on the map 346 published locations where blacklegged ticks had been detected and 198 locations where they had been searched for but not detected. Using statistical algorithms, Estrada-Peña asked whether specific combinations of temperature and vegetation data could discriminate positive sites (ticks present) from negative sites (ticks absent). A statistical model combining six of his variables performed remarkably well, predicting that ticks would be present in a particular location where they were actually absent only 6% of the time (high specificity), and predicting their absence where in fact they were present only 4% of the time (high sensitivity).

Given this perceived success, the next step was to create a map of habitat suitability for the continent, showing all locations where ticks would be expected to occur if they were able to disperse there. The map of suitable habitat for blacklegged ticks produced by Estrada-Peña's method (figure 25) was curious, because it included northern Alberta and the Northwest

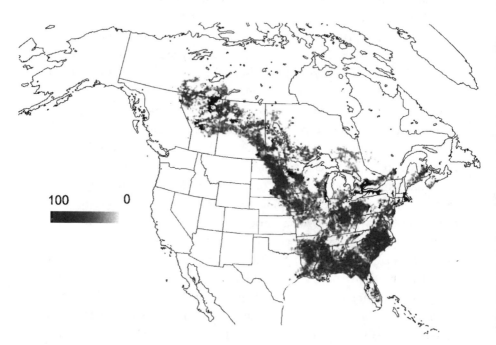

FIGURE 25. Habitat suitability for blacklegged ticks in North America as calculated by Estrada-Peña (1998). Reprinted with permission.

Territories of Canada in the suitable range but excluded east Texas and Oklahoma and much of New York and New England, where the tick is now known to exist (Dennis et al. 1998) (see figure 12 in chapter 3). One potential source of error was that only poor data were available for constructing the model. Estrada-Peña did not have access to a comprehensive map of the distribution of blacklegged ticks in the United States published the same year (Dennis et al. 1998). But I suspect that the major source of problems was the underlying assumption that blacklegged ticks currently occur everywhere climatic conditions allow and nowhere else.

In a more recent effort to produce a map of habitat suitability for blacklegged ticks, Brownstein and colleagues (2003) similarly mapped remotely sensed climatic data but departed from Estrada-Peña's procedures in several key ways. First, Brownstein's group made use of the map by Dennis et al. (1998) to discriminate between locations with and without ticks. Second, they included more climatic variables in their remote sensing data set—the mean, minimum, maximum, and standard deviation of four monthly ground temperatures (16 variables altogether). Third, they accounted for the likelihood that locations close to one another are highly similar in both climate and tick populations (*spatial autocorrelation*) and therefore not statistically independent. Fourth, they avoided assuming that the variables would be linearly related to tick populations and allowed the shapes of the relationships to vary in their statistical models. Last, they used field studies of the presence or absence of ticks in state parks that their model predicted would either support or not support tick populations.

The habitat suitability map produced by Brownstein and colleagues (figure 26) is remarkably similar to the Dennis et al. (1998) distribution map (see figure 12). Based on this map, one can conclude that blacklegged ticks in the United States currently occupy almost all the space that they can occupy. On the one hand, this is an encouraging result, because it suggests that the 16 variables used to distinguish suitable from unsuitable habitat work very well. In addition, their sampling of ticks at 20 state parks showed the presence of ticks in 15 of the 16 parks predicted to be above the suitability threshold and in none in the four parks predicted to be below the threshold.

On the other hand, the models used by Brownstein and colleagues (2003) raise some concerns. One is that the important predictor variables are quite hard to interpret biologically. For example, the best predictor of tick habitat suitability was minimum winter temperature, but the relationship was a highly complex sum of four variables raised to different exponents (*fourth-order polynomial*). This analysis (figure 27) would tell us

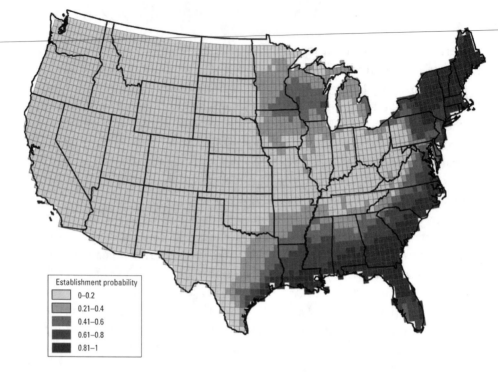

FIGURE 26. Habitat suitability for blacklegged ticks in the contiguous United States as calculated by Brownstein et al. (2003, their figure 3). Reprinted with permission.

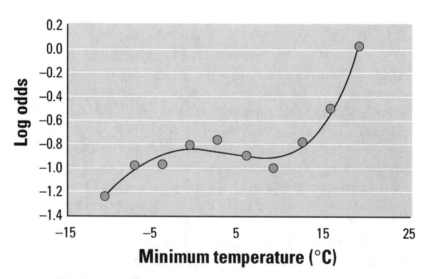

FIGURE 27. The best predictor of blacklegged tick habitat suitability in the model of Brownstein et al. (2003, their figure 2) was minimum winter temperature, but the relationship was a complex fourth-order polynomial. Reprinted with permission.

that very high minimum temperatures (>15°C) are best for ticks, somewhat lower minima (10°C) are quite poor, a little lower (~0°C) is better, and very cold (–15°C) is worst. Although such a complex relationship might in fact be correct, nothing we know about the biology of ticks would help us explain why. Related to this issue is a second concern, that the models do not specify any mechanism that might underlie a relationship between temperature variables and habitat suitability. In other words, the analyses are entirely correlational. This is not necessarily a flaw in the analysis, but rather suggests a caution that the correlations should be followed with studies of underlying cause.

Without understanding how climate affects ticks mechanistically, one cannot eliminate the possibility that the correlations, no matter how statistically robust, are false. For instance, Dister and colleagues (1997) used satellite-based greenness and wetness indices to distinguish between households in Westchester County, New York, with many ticks and those with few ticks. They argued that geographic (GIS-based) models built on these remotely sensed variables could be used to efficiently evaluate the risk of exposure to tick-borne disease at a fine scale. However, a follow-up study in Rhode Island (Rodgers and Mather 2006) found that these same greenness and wetness indices worked moderately well only in years when ticks were scarce and failed in years when ticks were generally abundant.

A third concern is that, although the model of Brownstein and colleagues (2003) does an excellent job of describing the temperature conditions where blacklegged ticks occurred in the late twentieth century, it has limited ability to predict where they will occur later, and tend to be conservative. This is because an expanding population by definition occupies only a portion of the range it will come to occupy, so the temperature conditions in its current range represent a subset of suitable conditions. Fourth, granting that the projected future distribution of blacklegged ticks is accurate, the consequences for the expansion of Lyme disease and other tick-borne diseases are not straightforward. As was discussed in chapter 4, blacklegged ticks occur in large regions with very little Lyme disease, because few of the ticks are infected or because population density is low (or both). For predicting disease risk, we also need to know tick abundance and infection prevalence.

The Brownstein et al. (2003) study led the way for later efforts to expand and improve our ability to map tick distributions onto climatic data and to use projected climate change data to predict where blacklegged ticks will occur in the next 100+ years (Killilea et al. 2008). Nevertheless, until the concerns above are addressed, confidence in these predictions will remain limited.

An alternative to correlational models, in which the presence or absence of ticks is spatially correlated with specific environmental variables, is the pursuit of causal relationships between specific environmental conditions and specific tick population responses. If the survival and numbers of offspring (*fecundity*) of ticks under various environmental conditions can be accurately described, one can then identify from first principles which combinations of conditions are likely to support tick populations, and possibly even predict future changes in tick distribution and abundance. This approach requires direct study in the field to assess the behavior of tick populations, and it also often involves laboratory study and use of remotely sensed data. The basic biology of blacklegged ticks suggests what some of these conditions might be.

Ixodes scapularis ticks are tiny, with larvae about 0.5 mm and nymphs about 1.0 mm long. Governed by the laws of geometry, such small organisms are destined to live with an extremely high surface-to-volume ratio. The relatively small volume and large surface area could potentially make these ticks particularly sensitive to extremes of temperature and humidity. A small volume means that the animal has essentially no thermal inertia and thus will be subject to the vagaries of ambient temperature. A high surface area means that water can be easily lost through the exoskeleton. Although inputs of water in the tick's diet (blood) are extraordinarily high, these blood meals last for only a week or two in the entire two-year life cycle of the tick, and for the remaining 98% of the tick's life there is no dietary source of water. While unattached to a host, the only source of hydration for these ticks is to dwell where relative humidity is close to saturation, where they can absorb water through the cuticle. Indeed, it's fairly easy to kill ticks in the laboratory by keeping them dry or under extreme temperature conditions. Subjecting larval blacklegged ticks to constant relative humidities less than about 90% will cause their demise within a week or two (Stafford 1994). Nymphal ticks are a bit hardier, surviving several months at constant relative humidity of about 85%, and surviving much longer at humidities somewhat below 85% if they are given approximately daily breaks in more humid spots to absorb water (Rodgers et al. 2007). Freezing a blacklegged tick to death is more difficult, requiring laboratory temperatures less than −10 degrees C (Burks et al. 1996, Ogden et al. 2004). Probably because ticks thrive when attached to mammal and bird hosts whose body temperatures can exceed 40 degrees C, it appears that the upper thermal limits to tick survival have not been thoroughly studied. One study showed that maintaining blacklegged ticks at constant temperatures above 32 degrees C prevented normal egg-laying in adults and molting in fed larvae and nymphs (Ogden et al. 2004).

In addition to causing outright death, low relative humidity can severely restrict the time periods when blacklegged ticks can leave the protection of being under leaf litter and in soil (high-humidity microsites) and can inhibit them from climbing vegetation to seek a host (Randolph and Storey 1999, Vail and Smith 2002). Low temperatures can also restrict the host-seeking activity of ticks, but perhaps more important, cold conditions can slow their developmental rates (Lindsay et al. 1995, Ogden et al. 2004, 2005). If low temperatures force ticks to spend longer periods in particular life stages, and if their daily probability of dying is constant during the time they remain in that life stage, then the result might be increased mortality rates (Ogden et al. 2004). However, although a slowing of developmental rate at low temperature has been demonstrated, a higher total proportion of ticks dying at low temperatures has not. But if temperatures are cold enough that blacklegged ticks are unlikely to undergo their complete life cycle in the usual time (~2 years), then higher total mortality seems plausible.

An additional, potentially profound, influence of climate (especially temperature) on tick-borne disease might occur if the seasonal timing (*phenology*) of host-seeking activity of larval and nymphal ticks is altered. Lyme disease owes its existence as a major zoonosis to the curious timing of activity of larvae and nymphs. Each year, larval ticks hatch and begin to seek a host in mid to late summer. As was described in chapter 2, these larvae hatch uninfected with *Borrelia burgdorferi*, and their only means of becoming infected is to feed on a host that is infected and efficient at transmitting *B. burgdorferi* to the feeding tick. By feeding in August or September, these larvae are quite likely to feed on an infected host, because the nymphs from the previous tick generation, which feed in May through July, will have recently finished infecting this same community of hosts upon which the larvae feed. These nymphs, many of which were infected, inject *B. burgdorferi* into their hosts. The bacterial infection then incubates and proliferates in the hosts, reaching maximal blood concentrations several weeks later, just in time for larvae to feed. If nymphs fed later in the season and/or larvae fed earlier, then the potential for efficient transmission of *B. burgdorferi* from nymphs to hosts to larvae would be disrupted. Indeed, this exact change in phenology, such that larvae and nymphs feed in the same season, is thought to contribute to reduced Lyme disease risk in parts of Europe and the southern United States (Randolph 2004, Jouda et al. 2004, Ogden et al. 2008a).

Blacklegged tick populations and Lyme disease risk, therefore, might be affected by climate by several distinct mechanisms. High and low extremes of temperature might both increase mortality and decrease fecundity, and thereby reduce population density. Low precipitation and relative humidity could similarly increase mortality. Warmer, less seasonal temperatures could disrupt the phenology that promotes tick infection with *B. burgdorferi*. Although the effects of very high precipitation and humidity on tick populations are poorly studied, the potential exists for natural enemies of ticks to thrive under extremely moist conditions. The most lethal tick pathogens and parasites appear to be arthropod-killing (*entomopathogenic*) fungi, especially *Metarhizium* and *Beauveria* species, and these fungi thrive under very moist conditions (Ostfeld et al. 2006c). So, it is possible that both high and low extremes of precipitation/humidity could inhibit blacklegged ticks. But how well do these observations allow us to explain and, perhaps more important, predict the geographic areas where Lyme disease risk will be high and where it will be low?

An innovative first attempt to incorporate the richness of potential climatic effects on habitat suitability for blacklegged ticks, and therefore on this species' potential geographic range, was made by Ogden and colleagues (2005). Ogden, Lindsay, and their colleagues (Lindsay et al. 1995, 1998, Ogden et al. 2004) had been studying blacklegged tick populations near the current northern limit of their North American range, near Long Point, Ontario. These studies and others provided Ogden and colleagues (2005) with data on how monthly temperatures affect development rates and activity patterns of these northern ticks. These researchers created a detailed model that simulated blacklegged tick population change by incorporating rates of survival, development, and host finding of all life stages as well as reproduction by adults (figure 28).

The model included 48 different parameters for tick vital rates and two for host availability (mice and deer), and perhaps because of this level of detail, the model was able to mimic naturally observed population fluctuations of larvae, nymphs, and adults reasonably well. Ogden's group then asked how tick populations are likely to respond to changing climatic (temperature) conditions. They incorporated their empirical observations that all tick life stages develop more slowly under colder temperatures, and assumed that the critical climatic variable was the average annual number of degree-days (days times average daily temperature) greater than 0 degrees C. A major assumption of the model was that the probability of a tick dying was constant each day that it was developing. The result of this assumption was that the longer a tick spends in each developmental stage,

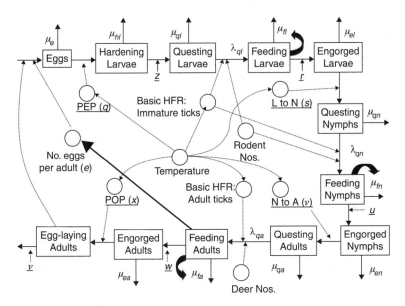

FIGURE 28. Conceptual diagram of Ogden et al. (2005) used to guide a simulation model of the effects of various climatic variables on survival, development, and host finding of all life stages of the blacklegged tick. Reprinted with permission.

the more likely it is to die. Their model indicated that there were extensive areas in southeastern Canada that are not currently occupied but that would be suitable for blacklegged ticks to invade and persist in high numbers. In later efforts, Ogden and colleagues (2006, 2008b, 2009) used similar models, combined with climate models that project future temperature conditions in Canada, to estimate that blacklegged ticks will dramatically expand their range even farther as the climate warms over the coming decades. The models of Ogden's group represent an emphatic early warning signal to residents and health care professionals in Canada that tick-borne diseases are on their way north.

These detailed, empirically grounded models have distinct advantages over the correlational approaches described above. Among these are clearly stated mechanisms linking climate to tick biology, critical details of tick phenology and host availability, and the ability to predict both tick abundance and tick infection prevalence (as opposed to simply predicting presence or absence of ticks). A major limitation of such models is that, simply by virtue of having so many parameters to incorporate, the probability of including false or unfounded assumptions seems quite high. For instance, the critical assumption that the daily probability of a tick dying is constant, such that more days in a developmental stage necessitates higher total mortality, is unsubstantiated. Similarly, the assumption that the relationship between temperature and tick survival is linear (a 10% increase in temperature means 10% greater survival, throughout the range of temperatures) doesn't allow for more complex relationships that might be more realistic. Another shortcoming is the inability to confirm that all of the variables important to tick survival and reproduction are included in the model. For example, even though 50 variables were used to build the model, effects of precipitation, humidity, and fluctuating host populations (independent of temperature) on tick vital rates are absent. Lastly, neither the correlational nor empirically based approaches are designed to compare alternative models each with different combinations of variables. For example, neither can address whether a model that focuses on total degree-days exceeding 0 degrees C performs better than one focusing on minimum winter temperature, or how those two models would compare with one that incorporates one or more temperature variables plus one or more precipitation variables. Given the complexities of the blacklegged tick life cycle, and the sheer number of possible chemical and physical (*abiotic*) factors that different researchers have posed as being important, it would seem that modeling and statistical approaches that compare different climatic variables are warranted. And, let's not forget that the ticks require three blood meals in order to reproduce, so potential host responses to climate must be considered.

It seems reasonable that climatic factors might affect the abundance of some of the vertebrates that serve as hosts for blacklegged ticks. In particular, white-footed mice might be vulnerable to extreme heat, cold, drought, or flooding (Lewellen and Vessey 1998). Working in northern Illinois, Jones and Kitron (2000) postulated that climatic variables might affect ticks directly and also indirectly if they influence abundance of white-footed mice. Monitoring ticks and mice over an eight-year period, they found that more larval ticks were detected after wetter (cumulative summer rainfall) years and during but not after warmer years (cumulative degree-days exceeding 10°C). Numbers of both mice and larval ticks were lower the year after extreme droughts. Interpreting these results is complicated by the fact that only one transect was assessed for tick and mouse abundance (that is, the study was unreplicated) and by the seemingly arbitrary selection of temperature and precipitation variables. These same variables were found not to correlate with blacklegged tick abundance, mouse abundance, or Lyme disease incidence at sites in southeastern New York State (Ostfeld et al. 2001, 2006a, Schauber et al. 2005). No follow-up studies have confirmed the importance of these particular variables or compared them to other climate variables.

Tick and mouse populations are difficult to monitor. Ideally, one must sample many different populations repeatedly each year for a good number of years, in order to piece together which factors, if any, most strongly influence survival, reproduction, and population dynamics. But if we're ultimately interested in whether climatic factors influence human exposure to Lyme disease, perhaps we can dispense with monitoring populations of mice and their reservoirs—the middlemen—and instead simply ask whether Lyme disease incidence in human populations correlates with climatic variables. Correlations between climate variables and Lyme disease cases might not tell us what mechanisms are involved, but it might be a good first step. The first such analysis for the northeastern United States that I'm aware of was performed by Subak (2003). Subak collated the annual number of Lyme disease cases reported in seven states— New York, Connecticut, Massachusetts, Rhode Island, Pennsylvania, New Jersey, and Maryland—between 1993 and 2001. She selected two climatic variables, the Palmer Hydrological Drought Index (a measure of summer moisture) and the average winter (December, January, February) temperatures for the center of the state or for the heaviest Lyme-endemic zone for the state. Because these climatic variables might act on any of the three host-seeking stages of the blacklegged tick or on mice (assumed to be the primary larval host; see chapter 4), Subak used the data from the same year as the Lyme disease statistics, the prior year, and two years prior, in simple linear regression analyses. For four of the states (Connecticut, Massachusetts, New York, and Pennsylvania), Lyme disease incidence positively correlated with the summer moisture index two years previously, but not with summer moisture in the same or prior year. Winter temperatures generally were poor predictors of Lyme disease cases. Subak's interpretation of these correlations was that relatively dry conditions in any given summer reduce survival rates of nymphs, but for reasons that are not evident, the effect of the reduced abundance of nymphs on Lyme disease incidence does not materialize that same year but only two years later, when the next generation of ticks becomes active.

McCabe and Bunnell (2004) analyzed largely the same data sets on both climatic conditions and Lyme disease cases and arrived at an entirely different conclusion, that Lyme disease cases in the northeastern United States positively correlated with precipitation during May and June of that same year, but not with precipitation in any prior years. (McCabe and Bunnell agreed with Subak that temperature was a poor predictor of Lyme disease incidence.) In contrast to Subak, McCabe and Bunnell divided the northeastern states into 38 regions, and so their spatial resolution was much higher. In addition, McCabe and Bunnell accounted for the fact that the total number of Lyme disease cases gradually increased during the 1990s, and incorporated this by *detrending* the data (analyzing the deviation from the trend rather than the actual numbers of cases). However, whether these different analytical choices led to the strong discrepancies is unknown.

Schauber and colleagues (2005) detrended the Lyme disease data (figure 29) and used states and a focal county (Dutchess County, New York) as the spatial units, and found that summer precipitation two years earlier sometimes correlated with Lyme disease incidence. However, the abundance of white-footed mice one year previously (this was measured only in Dutchess County, New York) was a considerably better predictor of Lyme disease cases, in both New York State and adjacent Connecticut, than was any climatic variable. All of the studies that have sought correlations between climatic factors and incidence of Lyme disease in humans have assumed that the climatic impacts are on ticks and only on ticks. None has examined the possibility that climate might affect human behavior such that the probability of encountering ticks is changed but tick abundance is not. For example, particularly warm weather in spring or summer could strongly increase the average time spent picnicking, hiking, or gardening—all potentially bringing people into close contact with ticks. If so, one might falsely interpret a positive correlation between summer temperature and Lyme disease cases as having been caused by climatic effects on ticks.

The results of these various climate studies are disappointingly inconsistent and confusing. Remote sensing studies of climatic factors that might limit tick habitat come up with different variables than do studies that ask what factors influence tick populations through time. No two studies that assess temporal changes in ticks or Lyme disease use the same set of climatic variables. Studies that choose to be explicit about the potentially critical climatic variables tend not to compare those variables with others. One of the key problems here is how to go about selecting climate variables.

Given the enormous number of variables that might be selected for analysis, it is sorely tempting to go on the scientific equivalent of a fishing expedition for the best variables. In this approach you have little idea where the fish (important variables) might be, so you simply drop your line (statistical model) into the opaque waters (data) and see if you get a bite (significant result). Essentially, you are indiscriminately throwing data into a big statistical model and seeing what comes out as "significant."

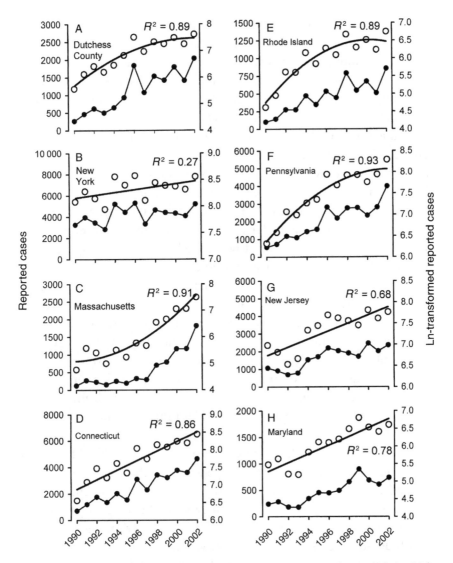

FIGURE 29. Reported cases of Lyme disease for some eastern states (open circles), which were then log-transformed (closed circles) to determine trends through time (curves drawn through the log-transformed data). These best-fit lines show various shapes, both linear and nonlinear, but all show a trend for increasing incidence through time. *Source*: Schauber et al. (2005). Reprinted with permission.

What's so bad about that? Why not compile a long list of potential temperature and precipitation variables for specific months or seasons in the current and several most recent years, and simply let statistical models tell us which ones best predict ticks or Lyme disease cases? There are two main reasons why this is a bad idea. The first is that any analyses that incorporate many potential explanatory variables (independent variables) require many more samples of the response variable (dependent variable)—namely, tick abundance, or Lyme disease cases—in order to arrive at trustworthy results. Given that the time series of Lyme disease or tick data are rarely longer than a decade, and spatial sampling of Lyme disease or ticks rarely includes more than a few dozen sites, this severely limits the number of climatic variables that can be fruitfully examined. The second reason is that the more independent variables that are included, the higher the likelihood that any statistically significant correlations are spurious.[1] Instead, it might be more productive to choose a small number of climate variables based on thorough ecological studies of tick population dynamics in variable climates. Unfortunately, given all the attention to the notion that, somehow, blacklegged ticks must be affected strongly by temperature or moisture, thorough natural history studies of blacklegged ticks have not been long-term enough or widespread enough to provide the necessary data on climatic influences. "Ecological monitoring" sounds dreadfully boring, and indeed, it is often the type of ecological study that is the first to have support withdrawn under financial or other constraints, and the last to get published in high-profile scientific journals. However, without widely distributed, long-term ecological monitoring of tick populations in varying climates, I think we have no way out of this conundrum.

Of course, any investigator who decides to monitor tick populations (or anything else) must choose what independent variables to monitor. For this it is critical to have conceptual or other models that generate expectations beforehand of what independent variables, alone or in combination, might be important. Designing a study so that competing models can be compared, rather than individual models being assessed using an arbitrary statistical criterion for significance, seems advantageous in this regard. Because we know that tick survival and fecundity are affected by the availability of various hosts as well as by climate, such models are unlikely to be useful unless they incorporate some host variables as well.

Temperature and precipitation are thought to act on ticks by killing them (too hot or cold or dry), by changing their behavior (host seeking or remaining quiescent), or by changing their developmental rates. But blacklegged ticks live in a physically and biologically complex environment in

---

1. When assessing whether two variables correlate, standard tests estimate the strength of the correlation (the "r" value) and call it "statistically significant" if the probability is less than 5% (1 in 20) that an r-value that high occurred by chance alone. But this also means that for every 20 correlation tests performed on any random set of data, one (5%) will come out "significant" by chance alone. This "significant" result would be false, or *spurious*. So the more tests you run, the more likely it is that you will arrive at spurious results.

which they have evolved adaptations to avoid or withstand inhospitable conditions. Heat and low humidity can be avoided by hunkering down under the leaf litter or entering soil pores that remain temperate, or by adopting a slowly metabolizing, resistant state (*diapause*). Both the abiotic conditions on the ground and opportunities to adopt avoidance strategies might be affected by the habitat type occupied by the tick. For instance, deciduous versus coniferous trees provide very different types of leaf litter, and slowly decomposing litter provided by oaks and beeches are quite different than more quickly decomposing maple and birch leaf litter. Sandy soils drain more quickly and remain drier than do clay or loam soils. The behavioral and developmental adaptations by ticks and the context of varying habitats have led researchers to seek associations between black-legged tick populations and various features of habitat, including vegetation, soil, and physical complexity. Again, though, this quest has been only minimally guided by specific, mechanistic hypotheses concerning what aspects of tick biology will be affected by what aspects of the habitat.

Throughout the Northeast and Midwest of the United States, tick researchers have repeatedly documented that blacklegged ticks are considerably more abundant in forests than in any other habitat type, including lawns, old fields, shrub thickets, and wetlands (Kitron et al. 1991, Maupin et al. 1991, Stafford and Magnarelli 1993, Duffy et al. 1994, Ostfeld et al. 1995, Frank et al. 1998, Guerra et al. 2002). In general, ticks are more abundant in fragmented patches of moist deciduous forests with shrub understories and are less abundant in large continuous forests and coniferous forests (Glass et al. 1994, Guerra et al. 2002, Allan et al. 2003, Lubelczyk et al. 2004, Brownstein et al. 2005; reviewed by Killilea et al. 2008). Although it is commonly assumed that, because of wetter, cooler conditions, ticks are more abundant in forests than in nonforests and in deciduous than in coniferous forests (see, for example, Lubelczyk et al. 2004), this assumption has rarely been examined rigorously. One exception to this was a study by Bertrand and Wilson (1996), who placed ticks in field enclosures and in nylon mesh bags inside intact forest, grassy fields, and the forest–field edge. The ticks placed in the forest and edge sites survived longer than did those in the field, which was hotter, drier, and more variable. Bertrand and Wilson also found that ticks that were free to seek better locations survived considerably longer than did those confined to nylon mesh bags. These experiments clearly help explain the causes of greater tick abundance in forests than fields. However, similar studies to compare tick survival and behavior among different forest types are lacking, and we don't know what might be causing the differences that have been observed.

Other researchers have mapped the spatial distribution of Lyme disease cases (rather than ticks themselves) and asked whether specific habitat features are good predictors of incidence. The spatial location of a Lyme disease case consists of the patient's street address as acquired by the health care provider who reported the case to county or state authorities. Therefore, attempts to determine localized correlates or causes of Lyme disease incidence are forced to assume that the patient encountered the tick that transmitted *B. burgdorferi* on his or her property. This might be a reasonable assumption in most cases, but it is very hard to evaluate. The main way that it has been examined is to ask whether Lyme disease patients tend to have more ticks, or more infected ticks, on their property than do neighbors who have not contracted Lyme disease. If one can demonstrate that risk is higher around the residences of sick people, then perhaps it's safe to assume that they got exposed while at home. Several studies have found that Lyme disease patients tend to have more ticks on their property than do nonpatients in the same community (Falco and Fish 1988, Maupin et al. 1991, Connally et al. 2006). However, it's impossible to rule out the possibility that the patient encountered the tick while walking the dog or picnicking in a nearby park, at a neighbor's barbeque, while at work, or somewhere else. The greater the fraction of Lyme disease patients who were exposed away from home, the larger the error in estimating spatial predictors of Lyme disease based on the patients' addresses. The size of this error is completely unknown.

In general, properties with at least one case of Lyme disease in the household are more likely to have forest on or adjacent to the property than are households without Lyme disease (Glass et al. 1995, Kitron and Kazmierczak 1997, Orloski et al. 1998, Eisen et al. 2006, Jackson et al. 2006a). But this is not a surprising result, given that blacklegged ticks are much more abundant in forested than in nonforested habitats. Associations between particular forest types and Lyme disease incidence have not generally been found.

Perhaps risk of exposure to Lyme disease is affected by factors that operate at some distance from the patient's residence rather than being determined only by what's inside that particular property. The survival of any ticks that are already in that property might be determined largely by highly localized factors such as the thickness of the forest canopy or understory. But recall that ticks get moved around quite a bit by their highly mobile hosts, so the number of ticks that wind up in that particular property could be affected by factors in the broader landscape. This observation has led several researchers to seek larger scale correlates of Lyme disease incidence in mixed landscapes. In what should be a familiar refrain by now, however, these searches are rarely guided by prior hypotheses based on specific mechanisms. An exception to this is a study by Brownstein and colleagues (2005), who hypothesized that areas in Connecticut landscapes with more highly fragmented forests should have higher incidence rates of Lyme disease, because fragmented forests promote certain populations of tick hosts, such as deer and mice. Brownstein's group rejected their hypothesis when they found that Connecticut towns with denser residential development and more highly fragmented forest had lower Lyme disease incidence rates than did more sparsely settled, more continuously forested towns. This result was curious, because Brownstein and colleagues found the opposite pattern when examining the distribution of infected ticks (that is, there were more infected ticks in more densely settled, highly fragmented towns). Brownstein's group selected towns as the spatial units for analysis because these are the political units in which Lyme cases are often reported, and they seem at first glance to be as good any other political unit. But towns, or counties, or postal codes—all readily accessible spatial units on maps—might be inappropriate for these analyses if the most important factors affecting Lyme disease risk occur at different spatial scales than these political units.

Two ways of addressing the potential mismatch between political units and biological processes are to conduct analyses at several different spatial scales and ask whether the results vary with scale, or to select spatial units that are more likely to reflect biological processes of import. Jackson and colleagues (2006a, 2006b) used both these approaches to examine correlates of Lyme disease incidence rates in a 12-county area in Maryland. They divided this region into 514 road-bounded landscapes, because movements of some wildlife hosts for ticks are inhibited by roads. Using roads to delimit the landscapes increases the likelihood that these sampling units are internally cohesive and at least partially ecologically independent of others. A limitation of this approach is illustrated every time one sees a deer, or mouse, or raccoon crossing a road—the roads are clearly not absolute barriers to animal movements. Jackson's group did not find that housing density or human population density affected Lyme disease incidence. They found that incidence rates were somewhat higher in landscapes containing many small forest patches, but the effect was fairly weak. Instead, the most significant factor was the percentage of all edges between habitat types that consisted of adjacent forest and herbaceous habitat, such as golf courses, lawns, or old fields (Jackson et al. 2006a). Lyme disease incidence rates were not higher in landscapes with more absolute amount of forest–field edge; they were higher in landscapes in which a higher percentage of all edges were forest–field edge. As far as I am aware, no biological interpretation of this result has emerged. Possibly a landscape with a high percentage of forest–field edge is more likely to induce people to enter forests or forest–field edges where their risk of encountering an infected tick is high.

So, what does all this tell us about how climate affects ticks and the diseases they transmit? It is not at all straightforward, and attempts to predict effects of spatially or temporally changing climate tend to fail. The rampant inconsistencies among the major studies, and the general lack of sound, biologically reasonable interpretations for those results that are strong, suggest that our conceptual models of how ticks respond to climate are far too simple. The ability to kill ticks in the lab by heating, freezing, or drying them does not necessarily mean that ticks in nature will be subject to the vagaries of temperature and humidity. We don't know whether tick mortality in the field is caused by the long, slow torture of suboptimal conditions—a little too dry, a bit too warm, for a bit too long—or by a single cold snap, heat wave, or deluge, or by too rapid a shift from cool to hot or from wet to dry. No matter which of these predominates, we don't know whether cold in January, heat in July, or drought in October is more important. And too intense a focus on climatic conditions can deflect attention away from the importance of hosts to tick survival and reproduction.

Although these are difficult problems, they are not intractable, and the importance of being able to predict places and times of high tick abundance and disease risk should drive us to invest in solving them. Field studies of tick survival under naturally varying and experimentally manipulated climatic conditions could be carried out along latitudinal or altitudinal gradients. Survival could be sampled after extreme weather events as well as more regularly. Such field studies can be coupled with spatial analyses of tick abundance or Lyme disease cases that compare the ability of different explicit, mechanistically based models to explain or predict the patterns. And, one must never forget the hosts—are they affected by the same factors that affect tick survival? Are they failing to transport ticks into climatically suitable areas, or delivering a steady supply to areas that can't maintain them? Are they abundant enough that they reliably rescue ticks from otherwise inhospitable conditions? Lastly, the human behavioral component is worth pursuing. Do hot, dry conditions in summer keep people indoors and away from ticks, whereas warm, dry conditions in spring do the opposite?

6

Questioning Dogma

IN 1981 PUBLIC HEALTH OFFICIALS NOTICED THAT A RARE AND USUALLY benign cancer of old people, Kaposi's sarcoma, had suddenly become more virulent and was attacking young gay men in New York City. At about the same time, a rare pneumonia caused by *Pneumocystis carinii* (now called *Pneumocystis jirovecii*) began to increase dramatically in New York, Los Angeles, and San Francisco, also largely among gay men. Something was causing the immune systems of these patients to fail, making them vulnerable to opportunistic infections. By 1982, similar syndromes were noted among people in Haiti, intravenous drug users, and hemophiliacs, who often receive blood transfusions concentrated from many donors. The different diseases were linked to a common cause and given the name acquired immunodeficiency syndrome (AIDS), even though the causal agent, human immunodeficiency virus (HIV), was not yet discovered. The demographic and geographic patterns that characterized the emergence of AIDS led to the rapid establishment of a paradigm: This deadly disease was spread during sexual contact between men and by blood-to-blood transfer; it had originated in Haiti and had been carried (probably by gay men) to major American cities, including New York, San Francisco, and Los Angeles. The discovery of an ongoing AIDS epidemic two years later in Western Europe did nothing to undermine the paradigm because many of these patients had a history of contact with gay American men. The notion that this was essentially an American, gay, urban disease stubbornly persisted for several years. Only in the late 1980s did the paradigm begin to be replaced by a more complex model of disease transmission and maintenance—by then AIDS was known to be caused by HIV, likely originated in Africa, was undergoing epidemics throughout central and eastern Africa, Europe, Asia, and Latin America, and was discovered to be transmitted during heterosexual as well as homosexual contact. Now it is known that far more cases of HIV/AIDS are transmitted by heterosexual than by homosexual contact and that the pandemic is massively more prevalent in sub-Saharan Africa (current adult prevalence 5%) than in North America (adult prevalence 0.4%). Under pressure from the public and from their own scientific culture to rapidly understand the source of disease, biomedical scientists had created an inaccurate model that had to be dismantled and then replaced.

Thirty years ago, no one would have thought that Lyme disease would become, by the turn of the twenty-first century, the most widespread and frequently reported vector-borne disease in Earth's North Temperate Zone. The enormous geographic distribution of this disease is prima facie evidence that the ecological conditions under which Lyme disease can exist are indeed broad. Nevertheless, at the time of its discovery in the United States, Lyme disease seemed to be a coastal problem that was localized in a few sites along the shores and islands of southern New England and New York. But why Lyme disease emerged where it did was not because these localities are optimal for the spirochetes, ticks, and hosts involved. In fact, sites farther inland appear to be better at sustaining Lyme disease. By the late 1990s, more Lyme disease cases per capita occurred in Dutchess and Columbia counties in New York's Hudson River Valley than occurred in coastal Connecticut, Massachusetts, or Long Island where the disease was first discovered (CDC 2008). Per capita cases in counties in western New Jersey, northeastern Pennsylvania, and northwestern Wisconsin are higher than those for any coastal or island counties except for Nantucket and Martha's Vineyard, Massachusetts (CDC 2008). Lyme disease emerged where it did probably because of historical accident (see chapter 2) rather than locally ideal conditions.

But, like HIV/AIDS, the place where Lyme disease emerged in the 1970s, combined with pressure for a quick solution, seems to have had a strong impact on how scientists pieced together the ecological factors involved in risk of human exposure to this disease. These islands and coastal areas are relatively benign, with warmer winters and cooler, wetter summers than one finds farther inland. Islands and coastal peninsulas also are ecologically somewhat peculiar, being characterized by lower species diversity than is typical inland (MacArthur and Wilson 1967). And sure enough, some of the initial studies of Lyme disease and tick ecology noted that adult blacklegged ticks were specialists on deer and immature ticks were found predominantly on white-footed mice. This result is not surprising given the scarcity of alternative hosts in these ecologically impoverished communities. The stage was set for a simple paradigm to emerge in the first few years after discovery: Lyme disease risk is closely tied to two host species—deer, which determine tick numbers, and white-footed mice, which determine tick infection—and is limited to areas with mild climatic conditions. Lacking a crystal ball, the scientists who first set out to unravel the ecological underpinnings of this disease could not have known that Lyme disease would quickly expand well outside this range of biotic and abiotic conditions. What is harder to understand is why the paradigm has persisted largely unmodified, in the face of contradictory evidence, for so long.

British ecologist Anthony Bradshaw is credited with coining the phrase that "restoration is an acid test of our ecological understanding." Ecological restoration is a rapidly expanding subdiscipline of ecology that is concerned with returning ecosystems to a close approximation of their structure and functioning before they were disturbed or degraded. Bradshaw likened ecological restoration to watch repair, in the sense that success depends on knowing the critical component parts, how they all work together, and what damaged the system in the first place. Failure to fully appreciate the complexities of these systems can lead to poor restoration or management outcomes.

A recent example comes from Macquarie Island, a World Heritage Island between New Zealand and Antarctica (Bergstrom et al. 2009). Macquarie Island was the home of an endemic parakeet and an endemic rail, as well as of penguins and many other seabirds. In the nineteenth century, first cats and then rabbits were introduced by sealing gangs who sought companionship (cats) and a ready source of food (rabbits). The rabbit population exploded by the middle of the twentieth century, reaching 130,000 rabbits on the 34-kilometer-long island, and their grazing caused the near eradication of all vegetation. In 1978, rabbit control commenced using a deadly flea-transmitted virus called *Myxoma*. About 10 years later, the rabbit population had been reduced to fewer than 20,000, and much of the vegetation had recovered. Unfortunately, the reduction in availability of rabbits for the hungry feral cat population led to massive increases in attacks by cats on nesting seabirds, causing the extinction of the endemic parakeet and rail and putting several other species in danger of local extinction. So, by the late twentieth century, the ecosystem was considered imperiled because native seabirds were being decimated by exotic cats, which, owing to the decline in rabbits, had little else to eat. Managers wanted to restore the nesting seabird colonies to their former levels and decided to aggressively cull the cats. In 2000, the last cat was shot. Unfortunately, the result of cat eradication was a population explosion of rabbits, which were no longer being controlled by *Myxoma* virus. The consequent destruction of vegetation throughout Macquarie Island was obvious even from space—satellite images document the rapid denuding of the island (Bergstrom et al. 2009)—and the remaining seabird populations are in imminent danger from habitat destruction.

Where did this ecological restoration go so wrong? It failed because the conceptual model of ecological interactions was overly simplistic. The endemic birds and nesting seabirds were affected both by exotic predators that kill them—a *top-down* effect—and by vegetation that protects nests from environmental conditions—a *bottom-up* effect. Overly abundant cats endanger the birds through a hyperactive top-down effect, so managers chose to alleviate this pressure. They failed to recognize that rabbits protect the birds when the rabbits are moderately abundant, by deflecting cat predation away from the birds. But rabbits trash nesting habitat when they're extremely abundant, a situation that arises when cats are removed. The general lesson about ecological communities is that the nature and strength of interactions between species can be indirect—that is, can be mediated by a third party—and often depend on which species are present and how many there are. Returning to Bradshaw, one could argue that environmental management of an infectious disease is an acid test of our ecological understanding of that disease. If we have limited success, or even fail, in our attempts to manage the disease, we should be willing to reconsider our ecological understanding of disease risk.

If blacklegged tick abundance is tightly coupled to white-tailed deer, then we should be able to manage tick populations effectively by removing deer or killing ticks on deer. The impacts of hunting or excluding deer on blacklegged tick populations are reviewed in detail in chapter 3; the bottom line is that results have been enormously variable. In some cases aggressive culling of deer results in near elimination of ticks, whereas in other cases strong reductions in deer numbers have had little or no effect on tick abundance. Counterintuitive *increases* in both tick numbers and tick infection with *Borrelia burgdorferi* have accompanied several deer removal and deer exclusion studies (reviewed in chapter 3). Why should such inconsistencies exist? One hypothesis favored by some researchers is that the removal of deer causes ticks that would otherwise have fed on deer to feed on other hosts (Perkins et al. 2006). Such an explanation might not cause

us to reexamine the basic paradigm that deer are the essential, or definitive, host of blacklegged ticks. Instead, we might simply have to adjust our
model somewhat to include the caveat that ticks can broaden their host
range when a preferred host is removed. Recently, some researchers have
been testing a device called the 4-poster that efficiently kills ticks on deer.
By killing ticks on deer rather than killing deer, researchers can avoid the
complication that ticks might change their host range if a key host is
removed. So, one might expect that the 4-poster would be even more
effective at reducing tick numbers than culling deer is. On the other hand,
using the 4-posters to strongly reduce tick populations would fail if adult
ticks already feed abundantly on other hosts, even in the presence of deer,
or if tick populations are regulated by nondeer hosts.

The 4-poster got its name from the two pairs of PVC posts that hold paint
rollers vertically on either side of a trough filled with dry corn (figure 30). The
corn attracts hungry deer, but to gain access to the trough and eat, deer must
position their heads between the upright paint rollers, which results in them
rubbing their head and neck against the rollers. The paint rollers are impregnated with an insecticide/acaricide, usually amitraz, which is extremely effective once deer have self-applied it to their necks and heads, killing virtually
100% of the ticks on deer (Pound et al. 2000, Solberg et al. 2003). The first
field study of 4-posters as a means of reducing blacklegged tick numbers was
conducted by Solberg and colleagues (2003) at a NASA property and one at
the Patuxent Wildlife Research Center in Prince George's County, Maryland.
Both sites were enclosed by fences, and the 1.2-square-kilometer NASA site
was provided with four 4-posters, whereas the 5.3-square-kilometer Patuxent
site had none and served as the control. 4-Posters were deployed in late 1995,
and ticks were monitored for the next three years. Examination of deer
anesthetized by sharpshooters revealed that 100% of ticks on deer were killed
by the insecticide/acaricide (in this case permethrin). Calculating percent tick
control as 100 × (average ticks at Patuxent × average ticks at NASA) ÷ average
ticks at Patuxent, Solberg's group concluded that tick control after three years
was 70% for nymphs counted on white-footed mice and 91% for questing
nymphs. Unfortunately, these results are hard to interpret because the study
had only one treatment and one control site (it was not *replicated*) and because
Patuxent, the control site, had considerably more ticks than did the NASA site
before the 4-posters were initially deployed, despite having equivalent densities of deer. It seems possible, therefore, that the Patuxent site was a better
quality location for ticks to begin with (for undetermined reasons), and that
site quality contributed to the greater number of ticks on this control site
compared to the NASA site.

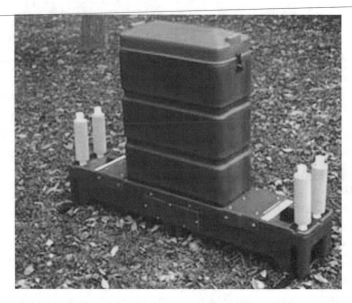

FIGURE 30. A 4-Poster feeder for attracting deer and applying insecticide to kill ticks. The central bin contains corn, which is accessible for feeding deer and other wildlife in adjacent troughs. To gain access to the corn, a deer typically must rub its head or neck against the vertical paint rollers (which give the device its name). When the paint rollers are impregnated with insecticide/acaricide, the deer self-applies the chemical. *Source*: American Lyme Disease Foundation (http://www.aldf.com/fourPoster2.shtml). Reprinted with permission.

A second test of the 4-poster, also in Maryland, deployed 25 of the devices in each of three 5-hectare sites and compared tick numbers with those in three control sites (Carroll et al. 2002). After five years of treating deer (1998–2002), percent control (calculated using the same formula used by Solberg and colleagues) for questing nymphal blacklegged ticks was 67%, 71%, and 77% on the three treatment plots. These reductions in nymphal tick abundance were statistically significant, and reducing nymph density by two-thirds to three-quarters is likely to have a strong impact on disease risk to humans. However, the fact that substantial numbers of nymphal black-legged ticks persisted after long-term deployment of these deer-targeted, tick-killing devices also suggests that substantial numbers of adult ticks feed on other hosts. In this same study, Carroll and colleagues found that the 4-posters produced 99% control of lone-star ticks (*Amblyomma america-num*), indicating that the considerably lower control for blacklegged ticks was not due to poor rates of insecticide delivery to deer. These studies suggest that blacklegged tick adults are not specialized on white-tailed deer (although lone-star ticks at these sites apparently are), so other hosts are important.

In fact, the results of the studies of Solberg, Carroll, and colleagues might underrepresent the importance of nondeer hosts for adult ticks. Researchers who have experimented with 4-posters (including me) generally observe that several mammal species, such as raccoons, opossums, and squirrels, are attracted by the devices and eat the corn inside (Carroll et al. 2008). It seems likely that these other hosts might self-treat with insecticide, enhancing the outcome for tick control. Recognition that adult ticks are more widely distributed across host species than often is appreciated could lead to the modification of these devices to more efficiently deliver insecticide to other host species. Instead, efforts to prevent access by these nondeer hosts currently prevail (Carroll et al. 2008).

A third study tested the ability of 4-posters to reduce ticks, this time in New Jersey. Schulze and colleagues (2008a) distributed seven 4-posters roughly regularly in a 66-ha residential community in Monmouth County and used two adjacent natural areas as controls. These researchers maintained 4-posters for two years (this study followed an initial 3-year period when both 4-posters and a mouse-targeted device, described below, were deployed) and counted numbers of both questing ticks and ticks on mice in the treated site and both control sites. After two years of this intervention, percent control of blacklegged ticks on mice was 40% for larvae and essentially zero for nymphal ticks on mice. In contrast, percent control of questing nymphs was about 87% after two years, with actual numbers of host-seeking nymphs on the treatment site about one-third as large as on the control sites. But again, without replication of treatment areas, rigorous interpretation of these results is difficult.

In August 2009 an entire issue of the journal *Vector-Borne and Zoonotic Diseases* (volume 9, number 4) was devoted to a series of papers describing the results of deploying 4-posters in Connecticut, Maryland, New Jersey, New York, and Rhode Island. Supported by the USDA, several research groups employed a common experimental design and measured associated effects on tick abundance in roughly similar fashion. Although considerable variability was observed among the sites, overview articles (as well as press releases issued by some of the authors) concluded that deploying groups of 4-posters generally reduces abundance of nymphal blacklegged ticks by about 70% (Brei et al. 2009, Childs 2009). Such conclusions need to be viewed with great caution. In all of the studies except that in Maryland, a single site was selected for deploying 4-posters, and ticks therein were compared with those in a single "control" site with no 4-posters. The researchers established this protocol in order to treat a *population* of white-tailed deer with insecticide and determine whether the

resulting *population* of ticks was reduced. This experimental design therefore involves only a single experimental population and a single control;
that is, it involved no replication. But statistical analyses of experimental
and control situations require that at least several populations be compared. In order to statistically analyze their data, the 4-poster researchers
had to assume that the dozen or more sampling plots within the single
experimental and single control sites were biologically and statistically
independent of one another. Such as assumption is analogous to the
following (admittedly absurd) scenario.

Imagine that one wants to test the hypothesis that eating green jelly
beans makes one's skin turn green. According to the 4-poster design, one
would recruit two people, feed one of them many green jelly beans and
feed the other nothing. One would then take pictures of dozens of different
parts of each person's skin—the nose, right arm, left leg, and so on—
treating each of those photographs as an independent unit for the statistical comparison, and then derive a specific probability that the difference
in skin color between the experimental and control person was due to
having eaten jelly beans. Such an approach is called *pseudo-replication*
(Hurlbert 1984), because many samples are taken from the single unit
(study site or human body) that was treated.

An additional problem with this design is the absence of a control for
the feeding of deer. Returning to the jelly bean analogy, if one found that
the bean-fed person was indeed greener, it could have been due to having
fed that person *anything*, not just green jelly beans, but one wouldn't know
this because the "control" person got no food at all. In the case of the
4-poster, it seems possible that deploying a number of feeding stations
might change the movement patterns of deer enough to alter the abundance and distribution of ticks irrespective of the insecticide. In order to
eliminate this possibility, "sham" 4-posters with corn but no insecticide
could have been used. In addition, in our jelly bean study, one would
clearly want to know whether the bean-fed person started out greener than
the control person, in order to interpret the effect of eating jelly beans, so
taking pictures "pretreatment" would be important. But in all but one of
the 4-poster studies, no estimates of tick abundance in the treatment and
control areas were made before the devices were installed.

Lastly, a hidden aspect of the 4-poster devices is that the corn therein
attracts at least several other hosts for ticks besides deer. Deer hunters who
deploy prehunt feeding stations to attract deer are widely aware of the fact
that corn and other deer baits attract raccoons, skunks, opossums, squirrels, and other mammals (figure 31), most of which can host adult ticks

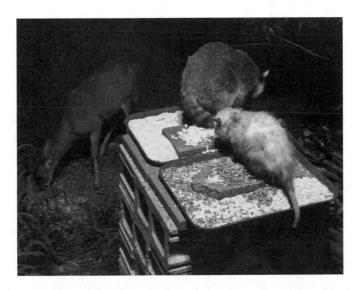

FIGURE 31. Photo of wildlife at a corn-baited feeding station used by hunters to attract deer. Note use of the bait by nontarget mammals and the deer in the background apparently being excluded from the food by a raccoon and an opossum.

(see chapter 3). Given the position of the insecticide-impregnated paint rollers next to the feeding trough, it seems plausible that most or all of these nondeer hosts might self-apply insecticide while munching corn. Although this nontarget application, if it occurs, would certainly enhance the efficacy of the device, it would also strongly alter our interpretation of the mechanism by which 4-posters affect tick populations.

Childs (2009: 356) interpreted the results of the USDA project as follows: "This study does identify the most vulnerable point in the Lyme disease natural maintenance system by clearly demonstrating the effect of targeting a single species, white-tailed deer, for reducing the abundance of infected ticks and subsequent risk of human disease." Although it is true that 4-posters *target* a single host, they might in fact *treat* several. As a means of reducing populations of ticks that might encounter and transmit pathogens to people, it seems that the 4-poster shows promise. But the design of the studies limits our ability to interpret the data.

In general, one would expect that treating a given number of deer with 4-posters would be more effective at reducing tick abundance than would killing the same number of deer. Killing deer indeed removes the ticks that were feeding when the deer was shot. But reducing the abundance of deer by hunting will probably result in many ticks encountering and feeding on alternative hosts. On the other hand, killing the ticks on deer does not allow for this possibility. Treated deer can continually attract ticks and kill them when they try to feed.

If blacklegged tick numbers are determined by deer, then attempts to control tick numbers by targeting white-footed mice with insecticides should fail. According to the dogma as I've described it above, targeting mice should strongly reduce tick infection with the Lyme disease spirochete but should have only modest effects on tick abundance, or no effect at all. The earliest host-targeted intervention aimed at blacklegged ticks and Lyme disease was conducted by Mather and colleagues (1987). These researchers took advantage of the tendency of white-footed mice to line their underground nests with insulating materials and devised a clever means of enticing mice to self-apply insecticide. They impregnated cotton balls with permethrin and deployed these balls in cardboard tubes on the forest floor. Sure enough, mice readily retrieved the insecticide-laced cotton to their burrows, and the numbers of immature blacklegged ticks on them were decreased by about 90% over the four-month study; almost three-quarters of mice had no detectable ticks at all. Unfortunately, the impact of these devices on risk of human exposure wasn't addressed by this study, because the researchers did not assess whether the abundance of questing nymphs was reduced. A follow-up study by Deblinger and Rimmer (1991) did sample questing nymphs after the deployment of 2,000 tubes in a 7.3-hectare site over three years. These researchers described a decline of host-seeking nymphs to near zero and concluded that the permethrin-treated cotton-ball device was highly effective. Unfortunately, their study design did not include any replication (there was only one treatment site) or any controls, complicating interpretation of the results. Nevertheless, these two studies suggested that tick control might be achieved by targeting mice with insecticide. But before the notion that mice affected the abundance—and not just the infection rate—of ticks could permeate the thinking of Lyme disease researchers, two better replicated, multiyear studies in New York and Connecticut showed no significant effects of these cotton-ball devices on questing tick numbers (Daniels et al. 1991, Stafford 1992). Despite the fact that rigorous field tests discredited the device's efficacy, it remains on the market for homeowners in Lyme-endemic zones.

A new mouse-targeted insecticide-delivery system was invented several years later and recently has undergone field tests. The newer device consists of a bread-box-sized plastic box with holes that allow entry by mice and other similar-sized mammals. Mammals entering the box—the "bait box"—are drawn to a food source but must navigate a tunnel to get there.

The roof of the tunnel contains a wick saturated with fipronil, a drug that kills arthropods (and is often used on dogs and cats under the name Frontline), which small mammals must brush by. Dolan et al. (2004) tested this device over three years on 300 properties scattered throughout an island near Mystic, Connecticut. They found that larval and nymphal tick burdens on mice within treated properties were reduced, respectively, by 84% and 68% compared to mice in untreated properties, and abundance of questing nymphs was reduced by more than 50%. These results are encouraging from the perspective of using mouse-targeted insecticide for reducing tick populations, but they are discouraging for adherents to the notion that tick abundance is closely tied to that of deer.

Perhaps more impressive than the reduction in nymph abundance caused by bait boxes was the reduction in nymph infection with *B. burgdorferi* from 24% on control properties to 8% observed on treated properties, a 67% reduction (Dolan et al. 2004). At first glance, this result would seem to support at least one part of the Lyme disease paradigm, that white-footed mice are the principal source of infection. However, it's important to note that, assuming only mice enter bait boxes, a 67% reduction in nymph infection means that about one-third of nymphs are getting infected by feeding on a nonmouse host (or an untreated mouse). Although Dolan and colleagues do not report on use of the bait boxes by other small mammals, such as eastern chipmunks and short-tailed shrews, my own experience with bait boxes demonstrates that these small mammals readily use the devices. In fact, internal examination of about 600 bait boxes my group deployed in Dutchess County, New York, revealed a few dozen that had been used as latrines by short-tailed shrews, with no evidence of use by mice. We also found clear evidence that chipmunks were frequent visitors of bait boxes. Consequently, it is difficult to evaluate the extent to which the reduction in nymph infection prevalence was caused by killing ticks on mice versus those on other small mammals.

A one-two punch was delivered to ticks by deploying both 4-Posters and bait boxes to a site in New Jersey—actually, it was a one-two-three punch, because an insecticide, deltamethrin, was also spread directly into the environment along forest–lawn edges (Schulze et al. 2007). The combination of these treatments resulted in reduced numbers of larval and nymphal ticks on small rodents by more than 90% compared to the two control sites. The calculated percent control of questing nymphs was 94.3%, but this number is somewhat misleading. Numbers of questing nymphs declined in the treatment area from 4.1 ticks before treatment to 1.4 ticks per plot three years after the control was started, whereas on the control plots questing nymphs increased significantly from 1.7 to 10.1 nymphs per plot. Because percent control is calculated based on differences between control and treatment plots, the unexplained increase in nymph abundance on the control plots had a strong effect on results, potentially exaggerating the percent control. Actual numbers of questing nymphs were reduced by about 65% over the three years of combined treatment with 4-Posters, bait boxes, and deltamethrin. When Schulze and colleagues removed the bait box and deltamethrin treatments, leaving only 4-posters to kill ticks on deer, they found that tick control was substantially weakened. This suggested that bait boxes directed at small mammals were the more potent control method (Schulze et al. 2008b). Effects of these control methods on tick infection with *B. burgdorferi* were not studied.

Jean Tsao and colleagues (2001, 2004) tried a completely different approach to managing human exposure to Lyme disease. They adapted the Lyme disease vaccine, which is currently used by veterinarians to protect dogs against Lyme disease, for use in white-footed mice. They first demonstrated that this vaccine, based on an antigenically active protein on the outer surface of *B. burgdorferi*, outer surface protein A (OspA), not only protects unexposed mice from infection with the Lyme disease spirochete but also clears the infection of those mice that were exposed before receiving the vaccine. After three injections with the vaccine, 99% of previously infected mice no longer transmitted spirochetes to feeding larval ticks (Tsao et al. 2001). The next step was to ask whether vaccinating a field population of white-footed mice in a Lyme-endemic zone would substantially reduce tick infection prevalence with *B. burgdorferi*. The follow-up field study that Tsao's group did in southern Connecticut (Tsao et al. 2004) was the first direct, experimental test of infection-is-caused-by-mice part of the Lyme disease paradigm. During an aggressive live-trapping program, they were able to vaccinate between 73% and 79% of the mouse population on their sites—a total of nearly 1,000 mice. Compared to control plots, vaccination reduced the percentage of infection in the next year's nymphs from 33% to 19% during 1999 and from 39% to 25% during 2002.

On the one hand, these results can be interpreted as confirming a potent role played by mice in contributing to the infection of blacklegged ticks. On the other hand, the fact that such an aggressive vaccination regimen resulted in only moderate (38% to 43%) reductions in infection prevalence suggests that nonmouse hosts are critically important to producing infected nymphs. Note that the results of Tsao and colleagues' vaccination study are quite consistent with the assertion by Brisson and colleagues (2008), described in chapter 4, that mice are responsible for infecting less than half of the infected nymphs in a population. Tsao and colleagues (2004: 18164) recognized this when they stated that "the results lead us to conclude that alternative hosts probably have a greater role in infecting larvae than most previous studies would predict. Accordingly, for reducing disease risk for humans, we encourage increased study of and emphasis on nonmouse hosts, including identification of other critical species for infection maintenance."

The experimental manipulations of ticks on deer, of ticks on white-footed mice, and of spirochetes in mice reviewed in this chapter do not support the paradigm that tick numbers are determined by deer and that tick infection is determined by mice. The last part of the paradigm concerning mild climatic conditions is somewhat more difficult to assess. With the exception of the unplanned experiment currently taking place, whereby humans have dumped sufficient carbon dioxide into the atmosphere to warm the planet, manipulative experiments of climatic effects on ticks have not been undertaken. However, a couple of studies have tested whether controlled burns can affect tick numbers. Because burning reduces vegetative cover and therefore makes ground conditions warmer and drier long after the burn, fire can provide an indirect assessment of some climatic effects on ticks.

But controlled burns have had underwhelming impacts on subsequent tick populations. Mather and colleagues (1993) burned a 15-hectare portion of a woodlot on Shelter Island, Rhode Island, in early April 1991 and followed tick responses. Sampling in June of that year, they found that abundance of nymphal blacklegged ticks had been reduced by 49% in the burned area. Not only did fully half of the nymphal population survive the burn, but almost twice as many of the nymphs that survived the burn were infected with *B. burgdorferi* compared to those on the unburned plot. Mather and colleagues argued that ticks that had fed on deer (and so were uninfected) were more likely to be killed by fire. The net result was that the risk of encountering an infected nymph on the burned plot was just as high as in the unburned area. Stafford and colleagues (1998) burned two sites in 1992—one was burned moderately in April and the other was burned severely in May. They found that June densities of nymphal blacklegged ticks were reduced by 74% (April burn) and 97% (May burn) compared to two reference sites. (Numbers of ticks on the burn sites and reference sites before the fires had not been determined, so the appropriateness of the reference sites as controls cannot be confirmed.) However, tick sampling later that summer and fall revealed that numbers of larval and adult ticks had not been significantly affected by the fires. In addition, Stafford's group noted that unpublished follow-up studies several years after the two burns found *increased* numbers of blacklegged ticks in the burn sites compared to controls, an effect they attributed to improved quality of deer browse and mouse habitat after the fires. Beyond the direct tick mortality apparently caused by the fire itself, no evidence supports the hypothesis that the ensuing drier, hotter conditions after a fire reduce tick densities.

Efforts to control ticks by interventions aimed at deer, mice, and microclimate—the acid tests described in this chapter—have generated highly mixed results and in some cases have failed. These failures have not been as spectacular as the attempt to restore breeding seabirds by killing cats on Macquarie Island. However, the results of these interventions underscore several essential lessons about the paradigm that Lyme disease risk is closely tied to two host species—deer, which determine tick numbers, and white-footed mice, which determine tick infection—and is limited to areas with mild climatic conditions. The first is that tick numbers might be determined more strongly by abundance of white-footed mice than by numbers of deer. At the very least, strong evidence supports the importance of nondeer hosts for both adult and immature ticks in affecting tick numbers. The abundance of nymphal ticks—the stage primarily responsible for transmitting pathogens to people—might be less tightly coupled to how many deer were available for adults of their parental generation and more tightly coupled to how many of last year's larvae found good hosts.

The second lesson is that tick infection prevalence is not tightly linked to any one host species, including white-footed mice. Several species are competent as *B. burgdorferi* reservoirs, and many others are not. Any larval tick that happens to feed on an incompetent reservoir like an opossum or a gray squirrel will not feed on a competent one like a mouse or a shrew; this is a consequence of the tick's life cycle in which only one blood meal is taken in each active life stage, larva, nymph, and adult. Therefore, infection prevalence of nymphs is a result of how the larval generation distributed itself across the entire host community.

The third lesson is that the capacity of ticks to avoid unfavorable climatic conditions, even during and after intense fires, effectively insulates ticks from tight climatic control. Moreover, the *indirect* impacts of climate and microclimate on ticks—acting through the community of hosts—might be at least as strong as those that act directly on tick survival. In either case, we have yet to characterize the climatic conditions that might regulate blacklegged tick populations. More effective means of controlling ticks and tick-borne disease will not arise until we replace the paradigm.

7

Embracing Complexity

Food Webs

IN MARCH 2003, PUBLIC HEALTH OFFICIALS REALIZED THAT THEY HAD a monster on their hands. A new contagious human pathogen, which had emerged the previous November in Guangdong Province, People's Republic of China, had spread to 30 countries and caused 7,900 illnesses, including more than 700 deaths. The disease was named severe acute respiratory syndrome (SARS), and the search for a cause commenced. A mere five weeks after the World Health Organization sounded an international alarm that March, the causative agent was identified as a novel coronavirus, termed SARS CoV (Rota et al. 2003).

New pathogens can arise in human populations by one of two pathways. The first occurs when an existing pathogen rapidly evolves into a form that is genetically and biomedically distinct, causing a new set of symptoms or having a new route of transmission. The other pathway occurs when a pathogen that circulates in a nonhuman species somehow jumps to humans. Phylogenetic analysis of the SARS CoV genome revealed that the new virus was not closely related to any other human coronaviruses, indicating that it had not evolved from other human pathogens (Marra et al. 2003, Rota et al. 2003). So a nonhuman animal (*zoonotic*) origin was strongly implicated at the outset and supported by the finding that animal traders and meat handlers in Guangdong had much higher rates of exposure to the virus than did the rest of the population.

By the summer of 2003, research groups began to aggressively round up and test various mammals from live-animal markets in Guangdong and adjacent Hong Kong, looking for the reservoir. Of the eight mammal species tested, masked palm civets *(Paguma larvata;* figure 32) were most frequently infected (6 of 6 tested), although the one raccoon dog *(Nyctereutes procyonoides)* also had antibodies to the virus (Guan et al. 2003). Partly because of small differences in nucleotide sequence between the palm civet and human viruses, Guan and colleagues were careful not to claim that palm civets were *the* reservoir. Nevertheless, Chinese public health officials declared a ban on all hunting, maintaining, transporting, and selling of masked palm civets, and much of the world assumed that the reservoir had been found (Shi and Hu 2008). (This ban was lifted four months later because of the economic toll it was taking on civet farmers and marketers [Normile and Ding 2003].)

Later testing of more than 1,000 masked palm civets from civet farms and markets throughout China revealed only a single animal market in Guangdong Province with infected animals; all other farms were completely free of SARS CoV infection (Kan et al. 2005, Shi and Hu 2008). The lack of widespread infection in civets began to shake confidence that this animal was indeed the reservoir. Confidence eroded further after the discovery that palm civets that had been experimentally infected with SARS CoV became sick with fever and lethargy. This was considered strong evidence against civets' status as the reservoir, because natural reservoirs of zoonotic pathogens usually don't show clinical signs or symptoms (Wu et al. 2005). A redoubled search for the SARS CoV reservoir revealed

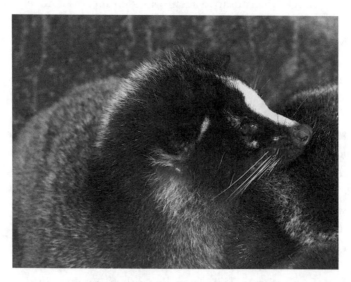

FIGURE 32. A masked palm civet, *Paguma larvata,* native to east Asia. *Source:* http://animaldiversity.ummz.umich.edu/site/resources/david_blank/ palmcivet3.jpg/view.html. Reprinted with permission.

that bats in the genus *Rhinolophus* (horseshoe bats; figure 33) were infected with, or produced antibodies to, a diverse group of SARS-like coronaviruses, some of which were closely related to those in palm civets and human victims (Li et al. 2005). This finding led Li and colleagues to hypothesize that horseshoe bats were the natural reservoir for SARS CoV, that these bats must have been maintained in particular exotic animal food markets in close proximity to masked palm civets, that the virus "spilled over" from bats to civets, and that civets amplified the virus and transmitted it to animal/handlers at the markets, who then transmitted it to other people in China, Hong Kong, and 28 other countries.

After publication of the study by Li and colleagues (2005), which advanced a plausible but largely untested hypothesis, the search for a natural reservoir essentially ceased (Shi and Hu 2008). Why did interest in pursuing the reservoir turn from hot to cold so rapidly? It seems that the public health community was deeply disappointed when several species of rhinolophid bats, rather than one species of farm-raised masked palm civet, were implicated as the main culprits responsible for maintaining the

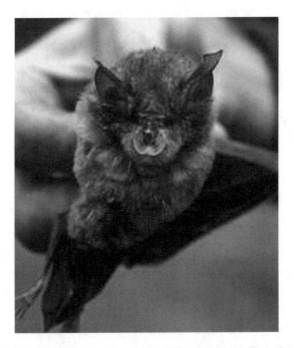

FIGURE 33. A *Rhinolophus* (or horseshoe) bat, named for the fold of skin around the nose. *Source:* http://animaldiversity.ummz.umich.edu/site/resources/ phil_myers/classic/rhinolophus_ferrumequinum.jpg/view.html. Reprinted with permission.

virus in nature. Commerce in palm civets could be banned by decree, but how would a government or international agency go about managing a bunch of obscure, widespread, cave-dwelling bats? The prevailing attitude seems to have shifted toward the notion that identifying the natural reservoir wasn't that important in the first place. After all, the SARS epidemic had been defeated not because of scientific knowledge of the virus, its reservoirs, its path of transmission from reservoirs to people, or the underlying causes of its emergence. It had been squashed by use of strict isolation of human patients—a centuries-old technique that predated the germ theory of infectious disease. (And isolating the patients was successful because SARS is highly contagious among people—an unusual trait for a zoonotic disease.)

Public health officials congratulated one another on such a rapid isolation, characterization, and treatment of a brand-new human pathogen, and SARS began to recede into memory, like a bad dream. But because the complex hypothesis advanced by Li and colleagues (2005) remains unconfirmed, we seem to have learned little that might allow us to anticipate and prevent the future outbreaks of SARS or other novel zoonotic pathogens that are certain to occur. The SARS epidemic is a success story only in the limited sense of response after the exposure, not in the sense of generating predictive power.

If the public health community wants to be able to anticipate outbreaks of zoonotic diseases like SARS, we need to know not only which species act as reservoirs, but also what factors promote or inhibit spillover to nonhuman animals and ultimately to humans. Emergence of SARS and of many other zoonoses (including Lyme disease) depends on cross-species transmission, which depends on the close contact between one or more reservoirs and one or more susceptible hosts, which in turn depends on the local distribution and abundance of these organisms, that is, their ecology. Yet, the ecological features (cave-dwelling? extreme crowding? food stress?) that might promote maintenance and transmission of SARS-like viruses in bat populations are unknown. The potential causes of spillover from bats into other mammals and of transmission among alleged intermediate hosts such as masked palm civets (crowding? poor diet? stress?) are unaddressed. These issues typically are not the primary concerns of the virologists and epidemiologists who admirably undertook the emergency actions to contain the SARS epidemic. They are the purview of ecologists, who, if the SARS epidemic is at all typical, will slowly progress in answering these questions during the mop-up phase extending a decade or more after the disease emerged, but long after public interest in and financial support for understanding the disease have waned.

One thing ecologists know about many infectious diseases is that the probability of pathogen transmission often depends strongly on the local population density of the host (Anderson and May 1979). Imagine a host population, let's say *Rhinolophus pearsoni* bats, in which all individuals in the population can be classified as either infected with the SARS CoV or uninfected and therefore susceptible to infection. Let's assume that the virus is transmitted directly from infected to susceptible bats, a plausible but untested assumption. The more infected individual bats, the higher the probability that the virus will spill over into some amplifying host or directly to humans. So, to anticipate outbreaks, we want to be able to predict the rate of increase in the number of infected individuals. Epidemiological models show that this rate is determined by the product of three parameters: the population density of infected bats (because they are the sole source of pathogens), the density of susceptible bats (because they are the ones that can become infected), and the rate of transmission between infected and susceptible bats. When these simple models are tailored to a particular disease, they can predict how small the population of susceptible hosts must be to drive the pathogen extinct, or how big it must be to set off an epidemic. So, identifying the reservoirs for a zoonotic pathogen is only the first step—to assess risk of an outbreak, one must also know what influences the abundance of the reservoir and any intermediate hosts.

Reservoirs for zoonotic pathogens, like all other organisms, live in food webs, which are groups of species connected by what they eat and what eats them (figure 34). An organism's position in a food web influences which other species it is likely to affect (which predators, prey, parasites, competitors, and so on), which of these species might affect its abundance, and how abundant it is likely to get. These interactions among species are also fundamentally important in determining which species are likely to share pathogens. So the ecology of food webs can be crucial for predicting population outbreaks of reservoirs and the probability of disease emergence.

Lyme Disease and Forest Food Webs

In 1991, I began a new study to address the role of white-footed mice in forest food webs. My colleagues Clive Jones, Charles Canham, and Gary Lovett had been monitoring populations of an exotic forest pest, the gypsy

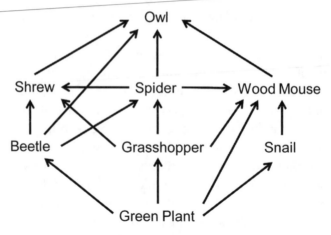

FIGURE 34. A typical food web, with plants at the bottom as primary producers, herbivorous invertebrates in the next trophic level *(primary consumers)*, invertebrate-eating vertebrates and invertebrates in the next higher level *(secondary consumers)*, and vertebrates that eat secondary consumers at the top *(tertiary consumers)*. *Source:* http://www.field-studies-council.org/urbaneco/ urbaneco/introduction/feeding.htm. Reprinted with permission.

moth, which had recently undergone a population explosion during which they had defoliated large expanses of oak forest, including the one where we worked at the Cary Institute of Ecosystem Studies in Dutchess County, New York. White-footed mice had been shown to be voracious predators on gypsy moths, especially the pupal (cocoon) stage, and we decided to test whether the mice might regulate the moths. Prior research had indicated that mice readily attack gypsy moth pupae and might even actively seek them out during the scant 2-week midsummer period when the moths pupate (see Smith 1985 and references therein). To test for regulation of moths by mice, we needed to know the abundances of mice and moths and attack rates by mice on moths. Clive Jones had been counting the egg masses that female moths lay each year—a good measure of moth abundance, so we had that base covered. To estimate mouse numbers in the forest, that summer we established two large field plots that contained a grid of live traps, which would allow us to repeatedly catch, mark, and recapture mice. Throughout the summer and fall, about 20 to 30 of the 242 traps on each grid would have a mouse inside on any given morning. By mid-October, checking the traps became hazardous, especially in the hilly parts of our plots, because the forest floor had become littered with acorns—sometimes more than 100 per square meter—and the acorns acted much like ball bearings under one's boots. The oak trees that

dominated the forest were producing a bumper crop of acorns, a phenomenon known as masting.

Sliding down one of these hills, I was reminded of a conference talk I
had seen the previous summer by my friend and colleague Jerry Wolff.
Wolff had been monitoring *Peromyscus* mouse populations in western
Virginia and had described how mice reach their highest peaks the summer
after a good acorn year. Acorns are highly nutritious, and some types can
be stored for months in underground caches, creating an excellent supply
of food overwinter. Mouse populations with access to abundant acorns
during winter survive well and can begin the spring breeding season
already at high density, whereas after acorn failure mouse populations can
crash to very low numbers (figure 35). This led me to anticipate that our
New York mice would be very abundant in the summer of 1992. The mice
did not disappoint, reaching a peak that August about five times higher
than in 1991. As our research group had predicted, not a single gypsy moth
pupa survived the rodent onslaught. However, perhaps even more striking
than the impact of this mouse plague on gypsy moths was the number of
ticks infesting the mice. The peak in mouse abundance in August coin-
cided perfectly with the peak in host-seeking activity by newly hatched
blacklegged tick larvae. Each mouse had easily 20 to 30 ticks on its ears and
face, so this quintupling of mouse abundance from one year to the next
suggested that tick populations might soar as well. Not only might the ticks
explode in numbers, but we expected that a particularly high percentage of
those ticks would become infected with *Borrelia burgdorferi*, given that
mice are the host most likely to transmit the spirochetes to feeding larval
ticks. It took almost a full year to test this expectation, because the larval
ticks that fed in August of 1992 are programmed to wait until the next
spring or summer before seeking a host for their nymphal meal. But it was
worth the wait—questing nymphal ticks were three times more abundant
in 1993 than in 1992, and they were 30% more likely to be infected with
B. burgdorferi (Ostfeld et al. 1996b, 1998). Altogether, the probability that
a person walking in the woods would encounter an infected nymphal
blacklegged tick was almost four times higher in 1993 than in the previous
year. Our group's monitoring of acorns, mice, ticks, and spirochetes has
continued to the present (19 years as of this writing), and the correlation
between fall acorns and next year's mice (figure 36), and between mice and
next year's nymphal ticks (figure 37), remains high (Ostfeld et al. 2006a).

What this means is that, in any area with endemic Lyme disease where
oak forests make up a significant part of the landscape, acorn production
is an excellent leading indicator of ecological risk of human exposure

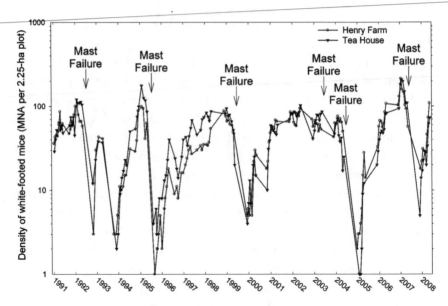

FIGURE 35. Population density of white-footed mice (numbers per 2.25-hectare plot) on two trapping grids at the Cary Institute, from their establishment in 1991 through 2008. Mast failures, defined as fewer than three acorns per square meter, were almost always followed by mouse crashes.

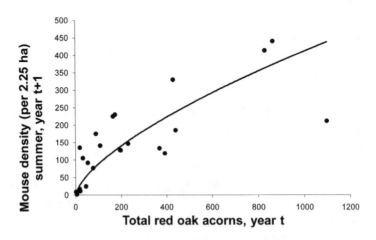

FIGURE 36. Relationship between total abundance of red oak acorns, as measured by seed traps placed in six large field plots, in the current year (year t) and midsummer mouse density in the next year (year t+1). Data are from 1995 through 2008.

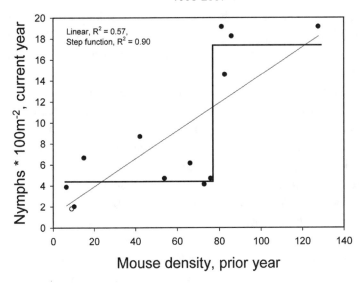

FIGURE 37. Relationship between mouse density (numbers per 2.25-hectare plot) in the prior year and nymphal tick density in the current year. Both linear and step-function curves provide a statistically significant fit to the data.

(Jones et al. 1998, Ostfeld et al. 1996b, 2006a). Simply by monitoring acorn production in local forests, one can predict how many infected nymphal ticks will occupy that forest two summers later. However, this observation couldn't tell my research group two things we wanted to know. The first was whether acorn-driven increases in ecological risk translated into acorn-driven increases in actual human incidence rates of Lyme disease. The second was whether the link between acorns and infected ticks (and possibly Lyme disease cases) was only a local phenomenon or whether the impact of acorns might be exerted regionally. To assess the relevance of acorns in predicting Lyme cases locally, my former postdoctoral associate Eric Schauber worked with Andrew Rotans (nee Evans) at the Dutchess County Department of Health and me to derive a time series of human cases of Lyme disease in the county. Dutchess County is well known for having maintained the most rigorous county-level Lyme disease surveillance program in New York State, and perhaps the country, so we knew that the data would be consistently high quality. We also knew that Dutchess County, like most other parts of the Northeast, had experienced a long-term increase in number of cases. This long-term trend complicated our analysis of the effect of acorns, because we suspected that the long-term dynamics of Lyme disease are determined not by long-term increases in acorn production, but by the geographic spread of infected ticks regionally and nationally from the 1980s to the present. Instead, we expected that acorn production affected whether a particular year was worse (more cases) or better (fewer cases) than expected based on the over-all trend. So we fit curves to the long-term data to describe the long-term trend quantitatively (see figure 29 in chapter 5) and then asked whether each year's deviations from the trend correlated with acorn production two years earlier. The answer was an unequivocal "yes" (figure 38; Schauber et al. 2005). We used statistical models to compare the ability of acorns versus some climatic variables (precipitation and temperature variables proposed by other researchers as important in Lyme disease ecology) to explain Lyme disease cases and found that acorns did a much better job.

To assess whether the predictive power of acorns extended to a larger region, we compiled data on annual Lyme disease incidence from seven states of the northeastern and mid-Atlantic regions. Our data on acorn production were limited to a 2,000-hectare site in Millbrook, Dutchess County, New York. Based on studies of tree seed production in other areas, we suspected but could not confirm that oak forests hundreds of kilometers

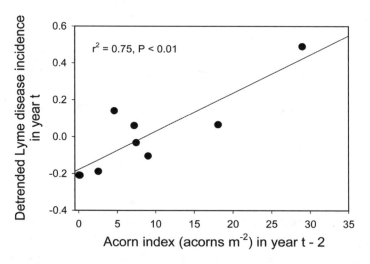

FIGURE 38. Positive correlation between the density of acorns produced by oak trees at the Cary Institute in Millbrook, Dutchess County, New York (acorn index), two years earlier (year t–2) and the number of Lyme disease cases reported to the Dutchess County Department of Health in the current year (year t). The two-year delay between acorn production and Lyme disease cases is expected from the life cycle of the tick, as described in the text. Based on data in Schauber et al. (2005).

away in nearby states might be producing acorns in the same years that Millbrook oak trees were. Again, we compared statistical models that included acorns in Millbrook as the predictor with models having several climatic variables measured in the center of the state as the predictors of the number of Lyme disease cases in that state. Models with Millbrook acorns performed as well as or better than models with state-specific climatic variables for Connecticut, New York, and New Jersey (Schauber et al. 2005). Not surprisingly, the predictive power of Millbrook acorns declined with distance; I have no doubt that local data on acorn production would provide greater predictive power for local communities than did the Millbrook data.

A simple food web of acorns to mice to ticks and spirochetes can provide an early warning system for Lyme disease risk. Nevertheless, some additional observations on these forest food webs enrich the picture and might ultimately increase predictive power. The first is that white-footed mice are not the only consumer species to respond strongly to acorn production. Our second most abundant small mammal, the eastern chipmunk, also eats and stores acorns, and chipmunk populations at our sites also increase dramatically the summer after a mast year (Ostfeld et al. 2006a). As described in chapter 4, chipmunks are the second most competent reservoir (after mice) for Lyme disease spirochetes and feed a considerable number of larval ticks. Although larval ticks feeding on mice have a considerably higher probability of surviving than do larvae feeding on any other host, larvae feed on chipmunks have the next best probability of surviving (Keesing et al. 2009). When we analyzed the first 14 years of our data on abundances of rodents and nymphal ticks at the Cary Institute, we found that models with only mice, those with only chipmunks, and those with both species combined performed roughly equally well in predicting next year's nymph population (Ostfeld et al. 2006a). With respect to their population responses to acorns and their ability to feed and infect blacklegged ticks, white-footed mice and eastern chipmunks behave quite similarly. In these processes, ecologists would consider them *functionally redundant*.

Shrews are the third group of small mammals with big impacts on blacklegged tick populations and Lyme disease risk (chapter 4). Shrews are insectivorous, however, and don't eat acorns or other tree seeds, so we don't expect shrew populations to grow in response to acorn production. However, because a high percentage of the acorns that drop to the forest floor are infested with the larvae of weevils, the possibility exists that mast years provide a pulse of food resources to shrews as well. Unfortunately, the live-trapping protocols that are effective in capturing rodents are not efficient for shrews, apparently because shrews are less attracted to traps baited with seeds, and we are unable to generate trustworthy estimates of shrew abundance to determine whether their population fluctuations synchronize with the rodents.

In at least one other food-web feature that might affect Lyme disease risk, mice and chipmunks are functionally redundant—both prey on eggs or nestlings of ground- and shrub-nesting songbirds such as veeries and wood thrushes (Schmidt and Ostfeld 2003, 2008). The role these ground-dwelling birds play in Lyme disease ecology is not well understood, but evidence is mounting that, although these birds are fed upon by larval ticks, they are relatively poor-quality hosts and kill most ticks that attempt to take a blood meal (Keesing et al. 2009). In addition, those larvae that do feed successfully from these songbirds have a low probability of acquiring a *B. burgdorferi* infection (LoGiudice et al. 2003), so songbirds function as protective hosts. However, it is possible that these birds transport larval ticks long distances during their annual migrations in late summer and early autumn, thereby increasing the spread of Lyme disease.

Research at the Cary Institute led by Ken Schmidt has revealed that exploding populations of mice and chipmunks after a heavy acorn year are

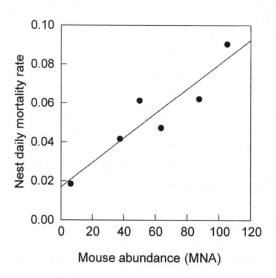

FIGURE 39. Positive correlation between the abundance of white-footed mice and the daily proportion of veery nests attacked resulting in the death of dependent young. Based on data from K. A. Schmidt and R. S. Ostfeld collected at the Cary Institute of Ecosystem Studies in Millbrook, New York.

particularly effective at finding the hidden nests of these songbirds. Attack rates on eggs and nestlings strongly correlated with rodent abundance (figure 39), so both fledging success and abundance of fledglings decrease with increased rodent abundance (Schmidt and Ostfeld 2003, 2008). Consequently, acorn production directly boosts availability of Lyme disease reservoir hosts (rodents) and indirectly suppresses availability of protective hosts (songbirds) the next summer.

But the effect of acorns extends beyond the next summer. Veeries and wood thrushes typically return in later breeding seasons to the vicinity of the nest where they were born, so the consequence of low fledging success in one year is fewer nesting adults returning the next year (Schmidt and Ostfeld 2008). In addition, those adults that do return the next summer (two summers after the mast) are subject to unusually high predation rates by raptors. The cause of this phenomenon is yet another indirect effect of acorns. During the summer after an acorn mast, when rodents are particularly abundant, barred owls, Cooper's hawks, sharp-shinned hawks, and other raptors prey heavily on rodents, and their predation rates on songbirds appear to be relaxed. During these summers, nestling but not adult songbirds experience high mortality rates. The rodent populations tend to decline rapidly from their peak (probably due to raptor predation), so their densities are particularly low two summers after the mast. The low abundance of rodent prey appears to cause the raptors to increase their attack rates on adult songbirds, reducing their reproductive output (figure 40). Only when rodents are neither very abundant (heavy rodent predation on baby birds) nor very scarce (heavy raptor predation on adults) do the songbirds achieve high reproductive output and population growth (Schmidt 2003). This "Goldilocks effect" (rodent numbers have to be just right) is a product of the acorn-driven food web and probably has an effect on Lyme disease risk. It appears that three different types of situations exist because of these acorn-driven food webs, although this hypothesis remains to be tested. One situation is characterized by high rodent and low bird abundances, which is expected to produce particularly high Lyme disease risk the next year. A second has low rodent and low bird abundances, producing low risk the next year. And the third has moderate rodent and high bird abundances, which will cause later Lyme disease risk to be moderate. Although rodent numbers appear to more strongly influence later Lyme disease risk, incorporating songbird abundance might increase our ability to predict risk.

One food-web feature in which mice and chipmunks are not functionally redundant, but that might profoundly affect Lyme disease risk, is their ability to control on gypsy moth populations. As good as white-footed mice

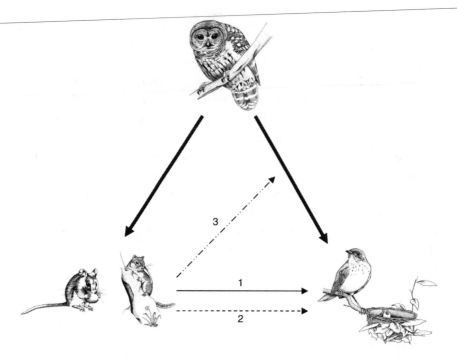

FIGURE 40. Simplified schematic of the interactions between ground-nesting songbirds (veery is illustrated), rodents (white-footed mouse and eastern chipmunk), and their shared predators (for example, the barred owl). The diagram illustrates the three interactions. The first is the direct predatory effect of rodents on songbird eggs and nestlings. The second is the indirect effect of rodents on songbirds caused by rodents boosting abundance of shared predators. The third is another indirect effect of rodents on songbirds caused by rodents changing the foraging behavior of shared predators. For more details, see Schmidt and Ostfeld (2008). Reprinted with permission.

are at finding and killing gypsy moth pupae, chipmunks are pathetically bad. Chipmunks do consume invertebrates and do forage on the ground and on tree trunks (where gypsy moths pupate), but for unknown reasons they don't attack gypsy moths (E. M. Schauber et al., unpublished observations). We know this because we have monitored the fates of thousands of both naturally occurring and experimentally deployed gypsy moth pupae over the years, and we have identified which predator species visit and kill them. For naturally occurring pupae, we place track plates around the pupation site, which provide us with easily identifiable animal tracks. When we experimentally deploy pupae, we attach them to a site with bee's wax, which leaves easily identifiable tooth marks after predation events.

Acorn-driven increases in mouse (but not chipmunk) abundance result in near zero survival of gypsy moth pupae, but during later crashes in the mouse population, pupal survival can be quite high (Elkinton et al. 1996, Ostfeld et al. 1996, Jones et al. 1998). But high pupal survival does not necessarily lead to an outbreak of gypsy moths. When moths are scarce at the beginning of the summer, even perfect survival will permit only a modest increase in population size the next year (doubling a modest investment generates only a small absolute gain). But if the mouse population crashes when gypsy moth abundance is moderate, or if mice remain scarce for two or three sequential years, then the moth population potentially can grow quite rapidly (figure 41). An outbreak of gypsy moths might at first glance seem unconnected to blacklegged ticks and Lyme disease. But when they reach outbreak levels, gypsy moths can defoliate vast expanses of deciduous forests (figure 42), and if the outbreak continues for two or more years, many thousands or even millions of trees can be killed. Because gypsy moths prefer to eat oak leaves, oaks tend to be hit harder than other tree species.

Gypsy moth outbreaks have several potential impacts on ticks and Lyme disease risk. First, because defoliation eliminates shade, the forest floor becomes much hotter and drier in summer, potentially causing at least temporary declines in tick abundance. Second, because masting requires that trees accumulate a large supply of energy over several years, a defoliation event is likely to delay acorn production by at least a year, altering the transient dynamics of mice and other tick hosts. And third, by causing the death of oaks, defoliation by gypsy moths can accelerate the decline of oak trees and replacement of oaks by maples and other species, which is currently occurring in much of the eastern United States. This last effect could have long-term impacts on Lyme disease risk by stabilizing tick populations that currently undergo fluctuations caused by highly variable seed crops. Whether tick populations would stabilize at lower or higher levels would seem to depend largely on which tree species replace the lost oaks. Maples, hickories, and ashes produce relatively constant supplies of seeds that are readily consumed by rodents (although they are much smaller and less nutritious than acorns), whereas birches and most conifers produce seeds too small for rodents to consume.

Rodents are by far the most important reservoirs for zoonotic pathogens worldwide (Ostfeld and Holt 2004). Zoonoses for which rodents are the main or sole reservoirs include Lyme disease, anaplasmosis, babesiosis, plague, monkeypox, bartonellosis, typhus, Lassa fever, leishmaniasis, Chagas disease, Bolivian, Argentine, and Crimean-Congo hemorrhagic fevers, and all the hantavirus diseases. Although the Order Rodentia has more species than any other order of mammals and is enormously diverse

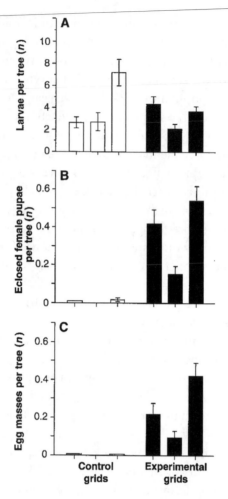

FIGURE 41. Results of the experimental removal of white-footed mice from three experimental trapping grids compared to three control grids. Panel A shows that mouse removal caused no differences in numbers of larval gypsy moths, which was expected because mice eat the later, pupal stage but not larvae. Panels B and C show the enormous, >30-fold increases in numbers of gypsy moth pupae and later egg masses on the grids from which mice were removed. *Source:* Jones et al. (1998). Reprinted with permission.

ecologically, rodents tend to share certain characteristics. Most either eat seeds exclusively or are omnivorous, eating, for example, insects and fruits as well as nuts and grains. They tend to have a high capacity for rapid population increase, owing to early age of maturity, large litter sizes, and short intervals between litters. Although predators are often important in regulating rodent population sizes, food supply is the factor most frequently implicated in regulating their populations (Wolff and Sherman 2006).

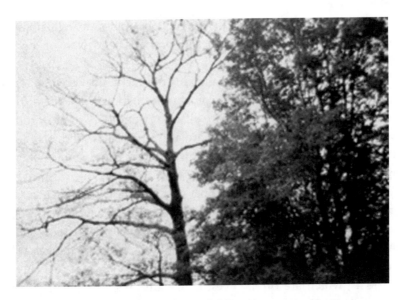

FIGURE 42. An oak tree in midsummer defoliated by gypsy moths. During moth outbreaks, millions of trees can be defoliated, and many can be killed, especially if the outbreak continues for two or more years. *Source*: http://www. ent.msu.edu/gypsyed/docs/forest.html. Reprinted with permission.

Studies of rodent populations from around the world are revealing that massive pulses of high-quality food driving secondary pulses of rodents are not unique to the oak–mouse–chipmunk–Lyme disease system (Ostfeld and Keesing 2000c). In arid environments of western North and South America, El Niño events cause unusually heavy rains that bring about population outbreaks of rodents, probably resulting from heavy seed production and increases in insect biomass. The resulting increases in risk of hantavirus pulmonary syndrome and plague have been linked to these resource pulses for rodents (Yates et al. 2002, Stenseth et al. 2006, Snall et al. 2008). Masting events by beeches and oaks in Europe cause eruptions of bank voles (*Myodes glareolus*), which in turn cause epidemics in kidney disease in humans caused by Puumala virus, a hantavirus that uses bank voles as the main reservoir (Clement et al. 2009). Another hantavirus that causes hemorrhagic fever with renal syndrome in Asia was linked to climate-driven pulses in autumn crop production and resulting outbreaks in populations of field and wood mice (*Apodemus* species; Bi et al. 2002). The biggest leptospirosis epidemic in Germany since the 1950s was linked to a climate-driven pulse in plant productivity that drove a widespread outbreak of voles, which are the primary reservoirs for the leptospire bacteria (Desai et al. 2009). These examples strongly implicate ecological interactions among species in food webs as drivers of zoonotic disease risk.

Whether pulses of resource availability or other food-web interactions played a part in the original SARS epidemic is unknown. The life histories of most bats (Order Chiroptera) are different from those of most rodents in some important ways, but there are also similarities. Perhaps the key difference is that bats have a much lower capacity for rapid population growth, given that their litters typically consist of only one offspring and they tend to produce only one litter per year (contrast with rodents, which typically produce four or more young per litter and several or many litters per year). But like rodents, bats can achieve extremely dense local populations, and locations where they group can move from place to place. Their behavior can cause them to group in very high densities—they aggregate in day roosts, which are often caves, and many species regroup at night in specific trees. Both day roost and night roost aggregations create the potential for massive pulses of pathogens that are excreted through feces or urine.

Changes in resources could potentially cause behavioral or physiological changes in bats that might contribute to disease transmission. Two other deadly viral diseases that use bats as reservoirs would suggest that underlying food-web causes are plausible. Hendra virus uses flying foxes (*Pteropus* species) as a reservoir and kills people and horses in Australia during spillover events. Nutritional stress of these bats was recently implicated as a major determinant of the probability of infection (Plowright et al. 2008). Similarly, the spread of Nipah virus, which uses different *Pteropus* species as reservoirs, has been linked to habitat destruction and hunting (Field et al. 2007). Apparently, not only resource pulses but also resource deprivations can elicit changes in reservoir food webs that increase zoonotic risk. For resource pulses, the mechanism—population increases by the reservoirs—is well understood. For resource deprivation, mechanisms have yet to be worked out.

As the acorn–rodent–spirochete–tick–human example illustrates, food webs can provide powerful leading indicators of heightened disease risk. We know that the risk of human exposure to zoonotic pathogens is affected strongly by how many reservoir hosts there are and by the closeness of reservoir groups to people, either directly, or indirectly through amplifying hosts. We have every reason to expect that knowledge of the food webs within which reservoirs are embedded would allow us to anticipate new epidemics. Whenever we have enough ecological knowledge to anticipate an outbreak, we can develop preventive measures to reduce rates of contact between reservoirs and victims, and we won't have to rely on the isolation and quarantine of infected patients after hundreds or thousands have already succumbed. In this sense, food-web knowledge can act as an ecological vaccine.

8

Embracing Complexity

Biodiversity

I DON'T HAVE MANY HEROES, BUT I COUNT DAVID QUAMMEN AS ONE. What's most heroic to me about Quammen is how he uses his boundless versatility as a self-taught scientist, journalist, and adventurer to teach the public about ecology and evolution. So, needless to say, I was delighted when Quammen wrote to me in 2007 to see if he could visit the field sites where we are studying ecological determinants of Lyme disease risk. He was in the research phase of a book on ecology of emerging infectious diseases, and his field trip destinations included Republic of Congo, Cambodia, Australia's Northern Territory, Gabon, Malaysia, Bangladesh, and the wilds of Dutchess County, New York. So for several days Quammen joined my field crew as we live trapped mammals and birds and collected blacklegged ticks in the forest fragments of Poughkeepsie and beyond, braving poison ivy, barberry thorns, and territorial dogs. These forest fragments sit behind school playgrounds, surrounded by strip malls or suburban yards, or adjacent to cornfields or golf courses. Some are tiny woodlots in backyards, and others are more extensive forested parks. Some have dozens of species of mammals and birds, while others have only a small handful. They might be somewhat less exotic and mysterious than Quammen's other destinations, but they're no less dangerous with respect to infectious disease, and they're no less subject to ecological forces.

As described in chapter 5, a group of small mammals are most important in producing infected nymphal ticks and increasing human risk of exposure to Lyme disease. Most prominent among these are white-footed mice, which are the most efficient hosts at infecting ticks with *Borrelia burgdorferi* and the best host for promoting tick survival (all other hosts we've studied tend to kill more than half the larval ticks that attempt to feed on them, as discussed later in this chapter). Next best at feeding and infecting ticks are eastern chipmunks. Shrews are the third most efficient reservoirs and feed large numbers of larval ticks, although we don't yet know how well shrews promote tick survival. All other hosts that we've studied are both poor reservoirs for *B. burgdorferi* and poor hosts for larval blacklegged ticks. Yet blacklegged ticks feed abundantly on essentially every warm-blooded vertebrate that spends time on the forest floor, irrespective of its quality as a host or its probability of infecting the tick with *B. burgdorferi*. Chapter 5 describes how risk of exposure to Lyme disease is linked to the abundance of mice, chipmunks, and shrews. But it also indicates that these three hosts don't begin to tell the whole story. Because each larval tick takes one and only one blood meal, every tick that bites some other (nonmouse, nonchipmunk, nonshrew) host will therefore not bite a mouse, chipmunk, or shrew. Our studies of Lyme disease, together with ecological theory, were telling us that our ability to predict the abundance and infection prevalence of nymphal ticks requires understanding the entire community of host species available to the tick population—that is, vertebrate biodiversity. The field studies that David Quammen came to observe were designed to examine how changes in vertebrate biodiversity affect risk of exposure to Lyme disease. The best possible laboratory for such studies is the fragmented landscape of Dutchess County, New York— the epicenter of Lyme disease in North America and perhaps the world.

To understand why biodiversity might be important in determining Lyme disease risk, it's important to remember the key features that characterize nearly all vector-borne zoonotic diseases, including Lyme. By definition, vector-borne zoonoses are caused by pathogens that use some nonhuman vertebrate hosts as reservoirs, and these pathogens are transmitted from the reservoir species to humans via the bite of a blood-feeding arthropod vector. For some zoonotic pathogens it is possible for baby vectors to inherit the infection from their mothers (*vertical transmission*). But even for those zoonoses in which vertical transmission is possible, the vast majority of infected vectors acquired the pathogen during blood meals from hosts (*horizontal transmission*) (Ostfeld and Keesing 2000a). So one key feature of vector-borne zoonoses is their strong reliance on vertebrate hosts for perpetuating the pathogen.

Another feature of vector-borne zoonoses is that the vector must be a *host generalist,* which means that it must be willing and able to bite more than one host species to obtain its blood meal. Although some species of zoonotic vectors feed from relatively few host species and others from many, all of them are host generalists to some degree (Ostfeld and Keesing 2000a). An example of an extreme host generalist is the *Culex pipiens* mosquito vector of West Nile virus, which feeds on dozens to hundreds of species of birds, mammals, and reptiles (Kilpatrick et al. 2007, LaDeau et al. 2008). At the other extreme are some flea vectors of plague bacteria, which tend to specialize more strongly on a few host species (Krasnov et al. 2008). For instance, some fleas of the genus *Oropsylla* are rarely found on hosts other than prairie dogs (*Cynomys* species) (Gage et al. 1995). Extreme host-specialization by vectors, however, can be very costly especially when the preferred host is wiped out by the vector-borne pathogen, which often happens with prairie dogs and plague. Consequently, even these pickier fleas are willing to bite other hosts, including humans (if this weren't the case, then humans would not get infected, and plague would not persist after the main host was killed off). Being a host generalist does not imply that the vector is entirely nonselective in its choice of hosts; it simply means that the vector species readily bites more than one (and often many) different host species. Even when the vector "prefers" some host species over others, the relative abundances of the various hosts is likely to influence how the vectors distribute their blood meals across the host community. For example, although some evidence suggests that *Cx. pipiens* mosquitoes tend to prefer biting American robins (Kilpatrick et al. 2006a, 2006b), these mosquitoes are quite willing to bite dozens of species of other birds, reptiles, and mammals (including humans) even when robins are abundant (Komar et al. 2003, Marra et al. 2004, LaDeau et al. 2008).

A third feature of vector-borne zoonoses is that the different host species vary in their *reservoir competence*, that is, in their probability of transmitting a pathogen infection to the vector during its blood meal. This is clearly the case for all vector-borne zoonotic diseases; some species are efficient at transmitting the pathogen to the vector during blood meals, whereas others are highly inefficient (Ostfeld and Keesing 2000a). To recap these three features, vectors tend to acquire zoonotic pathogens from vertebrate hosts, some of these hosts are more likely than others to transmit the pathogen, and the blood meals by vectors are distributed among various hosts that differ in their reservoir competence. Whenever these conditions are met, it must be the case that the composition of the host community (the species present and their relative abundances) available to the vector will largely determine what proportion of vectors gets infected.

If one more condition is met, then we can predict that high biodiversity in the host community will lead to low infection prevalence in the vector, and therefore low risk of human exposure. This fourth condition is that the host species that predominate in low-diversity communities tend to be the most competent reservoirs and, conversely, incompetent reservoirs tend to occur only in the most species-rich communities. Whenever this condition is met, vectors in a low-diversity host community will have a high probability of feeding from competent reservoirs and therefore of getting infected with the pathogen. Those in a high-diversity community will have a higher probability of feeding from an incompetent reservoir and of not getting infected. If the opposite were true—that the most competent reservoirs were found only in the most species-rich host communities and tended to disappear when species were lost, then we would find that disease risk is higher in habitats with more diverse vertebrate communities.

So, returning to the Lyme disease system, we need to ask to what degree these four conditions apply to *B. burgdorferi*, blacklegged ticks, and the community of vertebrate hosts for the tick and the pathogen. Regarding the first condition, we know that *B. burgdorferi* is acquired by blacklegged ticks only when they feed from infected hosts (horizontally, not vertically). Although one study found that a very small percentage (~1%) of questing larval blacklegged ticks were infected with *Borrelia* spirochetes (Piesman 1987), it is likely that these were not *B. burgdorferi* (J. Piesman, personal communication). Several other studies have found no vertical transmission at all (see Patrican 1997 and references therein). For the second condition, ironclad evidence demonstrates that blacklegged ticks feed readily on dozens of host species. We know that this tick species is a quintessential host generalist. The third condition is also clearly met: When we collect ticks that have taken their larval blood meal from different mammal and bird denizens of the forest, we find that hosts vary dramatically in their reservoir competence for *B. burgdorferi*, by more than 10-fold for some species versus others. So, three of the four conditions clearly are met. But what about our fourth condition, which, if true, would mean that more diverse vertebrate communities will present lower tick infection prevalence and therefore lower disease risk? Do the most competent reservoirs tend to occur in communities with the lowest diversity?

The different forest fragments that David Quammen visited with us are quite distinct in the number of different mammal and bird species they contain. In some we detect 10–12 mammal species and a few dozen bird species on any given day, whereas others might have only one or two species of each. The only entirely ubiquitous animal in this landscape is the white-footed mouse, which we trapped in every one of our 50 fragments (LoGiudice et al. 2008). The second most widespread species is the chipmunk. These rodents are quite resilient to human disturbances, such as forest fragmentation and degradation, and even thrive where forests are chopped up and otherwise damaged. Unfortunately, our live-trapping design is not optimized for shrews, so we don't know enough about these mammals to assess how widespread they are in urbanized and suburbanized landscapes. (Shrews have extraordinarily high breathing rates to support their high metabolism and are subject to rapid water loss whenever relative humidity is much below saturation. Therefore, on most days and nights they stay under leaf litter or logs and near their burrows, making them quite difficult to trap.) My personal experiences with short-tailed shrews that continually invade my kitchen sink, and a recent paper by Virgil Brack (2006), suggest that these shrews readily adapt to highly fragmented, low-diversity habitats, including urban and suburban environments. Brack describes a population of short-tailed shrews (*Blarina brevicauda*) living in a small flower bed surrounded on three sides by a large parking lot and on the fourth side by an office building in downtown Cincinnati, Ohio (figure 43). These shrews repeatedly climbed the three concrete steps to enter the office building, from which they were repeatedly

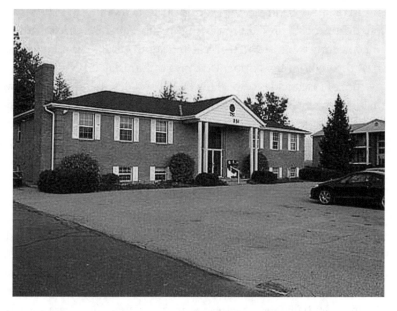

FIGURE 43. A parking lot in Cincinnati, Ohio, that was the habitat for a population of short-tailed shrews. The shrews regularly moved between the building and unpaved portions of the parking lot. These shrews, similar to white-footed mice and eastern chipmunks, often thrive in heavily degraded and fragmented habitats. *Source:* Brack (2006). Reprinted with permission.

removed. He also describes how short-tailed shrews invaded a garage in suburban Cincinnati where they attacked uncooked hamburgers that were being temporarily stored while a grill heated up. So, our field studies and some anecdotes confirm that the best reservoirs are the most likely species to dominate in low-diversity host communities. In contrast, the poorer reservoirs tend to be more sensitive to forest fragmentation, declining in abundance or even disappearing in the smaller fragments. In general, these incompetent reservoir species tend to be larger bodied, more carnivorous, or more specialized in their habitat selection. Species with these traits tend to require larger, uninterrupted habitat areas and are more prone to disappearing when habitat is chopped into little bits.

So high vertebrate biodiversity, achieved by preventing forest fragmentation, protects us from exposure to Lyme disease. Before describing in more detail the mechanisms by which this occurs, let's take a look at the general principles underlying the relationship between diversity and infectious disease. These general principles had their foundation in some ancient observations about the world's most frequent and devastating vector-borne disease—malaria.

In any given year, up to 500,000,000 cases of malaria occur worldwide, with more than 1,000,000 deaths (World Health Organization 2008). Most of these deaths occur in children living in sub-Saharan Africa. Although malaria currently is limited to tropical and subtropical regions, it formerly occurred throughout the temperate zones of Eurasia and North America. Massive use of insecticides (especially DDT) and destruction of many wetland habitats in which some mosquito vectors breed are largely responsible for the eradication of malaria from the temperate zone. However, some historians also credit the intensification of cattle production in parts of northern and western Europe for sharp declines in malaria that preceded insecticide use and wetland management (Brucechwatt 1987).

How would cattle production reduce incidence of malaria in people? Malaria is caused by metazoan parasites in the genus *Plasmodium*, which are transmitted by mosquitoes in the genus *Anopheles*. Most *Anopheles* mosquitoes tend to specialize on biting humans, but they will bite other mammals under some conditions. Similarly, the species of *Plasmodium* that cause malaria in people also tend to specialize on humans. This means that infected people are essentially the sole reservoir for *Plasmodium* parasites. New malaria cases occur when *Anopheles* mosquitoes transmit the parasite from infected to uninfected people. But when cattle production in parts of the British Isles intensified in the eighteenth and nineteenth centuries, it appears that increasing numbers of cattle in close proximity to villages and towns attracted *Anopheles* mosquitoes away from humans. Whenever mosquitoes bit a cow (*Bos taurus*) instead of a person, exposure rates of humans to *Plasmodium* infections declined. And because cows are inefficient reservoirs, fewer mosquitoes became infected in the first place. The use of cattle to protect people from malaria was termed *zooprophylaxis* (Macdonald 1957, Service 1991). Although cows are not typically thought of as a key component of biodiversity, the principle of adding species to reduce pathogen transmission applies here just as it does for Lyme disease.

The use of cows as a zooprophylactic measure against malaria was recommended by the World Health Organization starting in 1982, although more recently the WHO has backed down (WHO1991). The main reason that malaria zooprophylaxis using cows is no longer recommended is that, in some situations, cattle can *increase* malaria risk in people rather than reducing it. For example, in arid areas where sources of moisture for *Anopheles* mosquitoes are rare, cattle urine and feces can enhance mosquito survival and abundance (Dobson et al. 2006). Cattle housed close to people can also attract mosquitoes that would otherwise be more widely dispersed, essentially delivering them to the doorsteps of humans. In addition, if mosquito hosts are rare enough that mosquito populations are limited by host availability, then adding a bunch of cattle can increase mosquito density and malaria risk. And finally, if the proliferation of cattle as a source of protein for people causes the human population to increase in density, then *Anopheles* mosquitoes and *Plasmodium* parasites are likely to increase as well, given their dependence on people.

Therefore, whether adding a species (*Bos taurus* in our example above) increases or decreases disease transmission depends on some critical natural history features of the system. These include the effect of the added species on (1) vector infection rates with the specific pathogen, (2) vector abundance, (3) encounter rates between the vector and the main host (in this case humans), and (4) abundance of the main host. Zooprophylaxis as originally defined (Service 1991, Saul 2003) was a very simple concept, namely, that having a nonhuman animal near humans would deflect mosquito blood meals away from people, reducing transmission events. But when this simple concept confronted reality, it became clear that adding cattle could affect much more than just encounter rates between mosquitoes and people.

For malaria, Lyme disease, or any other vector-borne disease, we can use basic theory to deduce the dynamics of the system from two major activities—the loading of the pathogen from hosts to the vector, and the loading of pathogens from the vector to hosts (Antonovics et al. 1995,

Keesing et al. 2006). The loading of the pathogen from host to vector will increase with increases in any of the following: (1) the number of infected hosts, (2) the number of uninfected vectors biting those hosts, (3) the rate of encounter between uninfected vectors and infected hosts, and (4) the probability that those encounters will lead to pathogen transmission from host to vector. The loading of the pathogen from vector to hosts will increase with (1) growing numbers of infected vectors, (2) growing numbers of uninfected hosts, (3) increasing encounter rates between infected vectors and uninfected hosts, and (4) increasing probability of transmission per encounter. As described by Keesing and colleagues (2006), enhanced biodiversity will decrease pathogen transmission in any vector-borne disease whenever it reduces the abundance of susceptible hosts, the abundance of vectors, encounters between vectors and hosts, or transmissions when those encounters occur. Conversely, enhanced biodiversity will *increase* pathogen transmission and disease risk whenever it increases those four variables. Zooprophylaxis by adding cattle was originally envisaged as reducing encounter rates between infected mosquitoes and people, yet now we see that adding cattle can operate in several other ways, with a net effect that's hard to predict without specific natural history knowledge.

Whenever increasing biodiversity causes a decrease in pathogen transmission or disease risk, we call this the *dilution effect* (VanBuskirk and Ostfeld 1995, Ostfeld and Keesing 2000b). The opposite—increased pathogen transmission caused by increasing biodiversity—is called an *amplification effect* (Keesing et al. 2006). Unlike zooprophylaxis, which invokes a reduced encounter rate between vectors and human victims, the dilution effect does not imply a specific mechanism. Rather, the dilution effect describes a phenomenon that can be caused by one or more of several specific mechanisms. Exploration of theoretical models of epidemiology (Keesing et al. 2006) identified at least six possible mechanisms by which increasing biodiversity can reduce pathogen transmission. It appears that three of these are widespread and powerful among the vector-borne diseases, although the other three have rarely if ever been addressed and might operate as well. Before describing how each of the three mechanisms operates in Lyme disease, let me first discuss them in more general terms.

Imagine a simple vector-borne zoonotic system consisting of three species—the pathogen, one vector, and one vertebrate reservoir host. Both vectors and reservoirs are divided into those that are infected and those that are uninfected. Uninfected reservoirs get infected when they are bitten by an infected vector, and uninfected vectors get infected when they bite an infected reservoir host. Now imagine that we add a second vertebrate species to the system. If this new species preys upon or competes for resources with the reservoir species, then its addition will cause a decline in abundance of the reservoir. Because a decline in the density of the reservoir will reduce the opportunities for pathogen transmission from reservoir to vector and from vector to reservoir (see, for example, Anderson and May 1979, 1981, Ostfeld and Holt 2004), adding this new vertebrate to this hypothetical system will decrease disease risk via *host regulation* (Keesing et al. 2006).

Now imagine that the added vertebrate (which we're assuming is either a predator on or competitor with the reservoir) causes the reservoir host to become more sedentary as a way to avoid predation and competition (reduced home range size in the presence of predators and competitors is common). Reduced ranging behavior by the reservoir host will make it less likely to encounter a vector, thereby reducing opportunities for pathogen transmission from vector to host and from host to vector. Keesing and colleagues (2006) called this *encounter reduction*. Encounters can also be reduced if the added vertebrate acts as a secondary host for the vector. In this case, the new host species will attract vectors that would otherwise have had only the reservoir host to feed on, so encounter rates are reduced between the vector and the reservoir host. (Note that this specific type of encounter reduction defines zooprophylaxis.) Finally, imagine a situation in which the added vertebrate species can act as a host for the vector but is a poorer quality host, such that vectors feeding on the new host species are less likely to survive or reproduce than are those that feed on the reservoir host. In this case, the increase in diversity accomplished by adding the new vertebrate species will regulate the size of the vector population (*vector regulation*; Keesing et al. 2006).

Notice that these hypothetical models make some assumptions about the way that the new, added species interacts with the reservoir host and the vector. In theory, it's equally likely that the added species would *increase* abundance of the reservoir host (for example, if it is a prey rather than predator or competitor), or it might *increase* encounter rates between the vector and reservoir host, or it might *increase* abundance of the vector (if it adds a blood meal source for a vector that is limited by blood meal sources). If the added species has any of these effects, it might increase disease risk by an amplification effect. So it's important to return from the hypothetical to the real world to ask about the impact of additional species in more diverse communities on abundance of the main reservoir, encounter rates between the main reservoir and the vector, and the survival and abundance of vectors.

First, let's ask about the impact of biodiversity on abundance of reservoir hosts. In chapter 7 I described the importance of a key food source—acorns—on the abundance of the most efficient Lyme disease reservoir, the white-footed mouse. Our long-term studies in Millbrook, New York, show that about 60% of the year-to-year variation in summer density of white-footed mice is explained by the number of acorns produced by local oak trees the prior autumn. These observations indicate that 40% of the variation in mouse abundance in oak forests remains to be explained. And mice live in many other habitat types besides oak forests—they occur in essentially every terrestrial habitat within their geographic range (chapter 4), from old growth, pristine forests to degraded woodlots to shrub thickets to suburban kitchens. Because some of these habitats have no acorns at all, we must look to other sources of mouse population regulation. To test the hypothesis that high vertebrate biodiversity regulates populations of white-footed mice (host regulation), my colleagues and I established 40 field sites in New York, New Jersey, and Connecticut where Lyme disease is endemic. These sites consisted of forest fragments of different sizes, typically between 1 and about 10 hectares, and in various landscape contexts— some were in suburban developments, others in agricultural fields, yet others surrounded by strip malls. The sites also varied substantially in the type of forest they supported, with quite different tree species and understory species. We used standard mark–recapture techniques with live traps to estimate the abundance of white-footed mice in each of the sites. We also used several other sizes of live traps, stationary cameras that are triggered when a sensor detects motion, scat (feces) surveys, and watching/listening stations for birds to compile lists of all the other mammal and bird species that occupy each of the sites. These were our biodiversity surveys.

We found that the lower the diversity (number of species) of predatory mammals and birds, the greater the population density of white-footed mice among sites (LoGiudice et al. 2008). The scatter in the data is considerable (figure 44) and was expected given that the sites differed so strongly in many features that might affect habitat quality and accessibility for mice. Nevertheless, despite this statistical "noise," high predator diversity still constituted a clear statistical "signal" reducing average mouse abundance. The host-regulation mode of dilution is supported in the Lyme disease system.

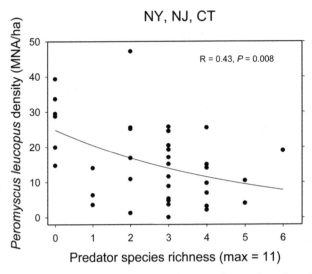

FIGURE 44. Significant negative correlation between the number of species of predatory mammals and birds in a forest patch and the population density of white-footed mice in that patch. The data set consists of 40 forest fragments in New York, New Jersey, and Connecticut that were intensively studied for their vertebrate faunas.

Next we can ask whether increases in the abundance of nonmouse hosts change encounter rates between tick vectors and mice. To do this most rigorously, my colleague Jesse Brunner and I (Brunner and Ostfeld 2008) used our long-term data from our Millbrook sites to ask what variables affect the number of larval ticks that feed on individual white-footed mice. Here we assumed that encounter rates between ticks and mice are reflected in the numbers of ticks we count on those mice in the field. In theory, many different factors can influence how many larval ticks feed on the average mouse in a Lyme disease zone—for example, the site where the mouse lived, the year it lived, its sex or age or body mass, or how many larval ticks were crawling about on the forest floor. Because we had such an enormous data set at our disposal (>23,000 capture records of >10,200 mice over 14 years), Brunner and I were able to construct a series of statistical models, with each model using a different combination of potential causal factors. We then used information-theoretic approaches to ask which of the models are best supported by the data. We found that many factors influence the average number of larval ticks on a white-footed mouse. Mice are more heavily infested in some sites than others and in some years than others, for reasons we don't yet understand. Some other relationships are easier to understand. Mice in sites and years with more questing larvae have more ticks attached; males have more ticks than do females (more parasites on males than females is quite common and is probably caused by less fastidious grooming and larger home ranges of males); bigger mice have more ticks than do littler mice.

But the most potent factor that reduced the number of larval ticks attached to mice was an increase in the number of chipmunks on the plot (figure 45). As the density of chipmunks varied from near zero to 80 animals per plot, the average number of larvae on mice dropped by a whopping 20 ticks! This observation strongly supports the hypothesis that increases in availability of nonmouse hosts deflect tick meals away from mice and thereby decrease the average burden of larval ticks per mouse. We interpret this as strong support for the encounter-reduction mechanism of the dilution effect.

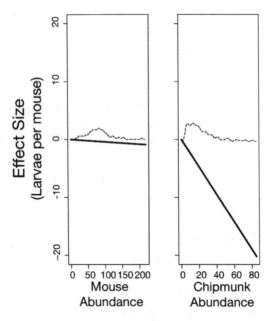

FIGURE 45. The effect of naturally varying abundances of white-footed mice and eastern chipmunks on the average number of larval ticks on individual mice (solid, straight lines; dashed lines are frequency distributions). Data are from six plots monitored over 14 years at Cary Institute of Ecosystem Studies in Millbrook, New York. The abundance of mice in a particular field plot had little effect on the average tick burden on mice (left panel), whereas the abundance of chipmunks had a huge effect, strongly reducing the average number of larval ticks on mice. These data strongly suggest that increasing availability of nonmouse hosts can deflect tick meals away from mice. For more details, see Brunner and Ostfeld (2008).

Finally, we can ask how an increase in host biodiversity affects the abundance of tick vectors. If all host species are identical in their quality as hosts for larval ticks, then the diversity in the host community will not affect tick populations, because species identity and community composition will not affect tick survival. On the other hand, if some host species are high-quality and others poor hosts, then the availability of each host species matters to tick survival and population dynamics. There are several possible mechanisms by which hosts can affect tick fitness. Hosts might differ in the quantity or quality of blood that ticks are able to imbibe, leading to differential success in molting to the next stage (LoGiudice et al. 2003) or differing overwinter survival of newly molted ticks (my lab is currently assessing this mechanism). Perhaps the most obvious mechanism, though, is the probability that a larval tick will survive its attempt to feed from each species of host.

Once they encounter a host, larval ticks will crawl around the skin, fur, feathers, or scales of the host sometimes for many hours before selecting a site to embed their mouth parts. Once they've chosen a spot, they remain attached and immobile for several days. During both the preattachment and attachment phases, ticks are quite vulnerable to routine grooming by the host, and ticks can be injured or killed when the host scratches, bites, or licks the tick off. While the tick's mouth parts are embedded in the host's skin, immune responses by the host to salivary and other antigens can cause an inflammation that might stimulate grooming. In some cases, the immune response to tick salivary antigens is strong enough to kill the tick outright, without dislodging or eating it (Zeidner et al. 1997, Burke et al. 2005, Muller-Doblies et al. 2007). (It is noteworthy that antibody responses by hosts to ticks, and not to pathogens within ticks, are now considered the most promising candidates for vaccine development against tick-borne diseases.) The fact that tick saliva contains such a rich pharmacopeia of anti-inflammatories, analgesics, anticoagulants, and antihistamines (Ribeiro et al. 2006) suggests that self-defense by hosts, including grooming, has been critically important in tick evolution. Ticks and hosts appear to be engaged in an evolutionary arms race, in which ticks evolve to evade detection by hosts, and hosts evolve to detect and destroy these parasites.

Our recent research shows that some host species are much better at detecting and destroying ticks than are others (Keesing et al. 2009). We selected six different host species that our evidence shows are typically heavily parasitized by ticks but that vary in features important to Lyme disease ecology—reservoir competence, average tick burdens, body size,

and abundance. The six species were white-footed mice, eastern chipmunks, eastern gray squirrels, Virginia opossums, gray catbirds, and
veeries. Using live traps for mammals and mist nets for birds, we went out
to the field in August (the peak of larval tick activity) and captured representative individuals of each species and retrieved them to the lab. We held
them for three days in wire mesh cages to let all the naturally occurring
larval ticks drop off into pans of water below. We then placed 100 active
larval blacklegged ticks on each individual host, treating each host species
the same, and after four hours in a holding chamber, we returned the host
to its wire mesh cage. Over the next four days we carefully tracked the fates
of all 100 ticks placed on each host.

The results were dramatic. On average, 50% of the larval ticks we
placed on white-footed mice survived to eat their fill (*repletion*) and
dropped off the host in an engorged state. In contrast, only 3.5% of the
larval ticks place on opossums survived to repletion, with almost all the
rest being killed and consumed by the host. Numbers for chipmunks,
squirrels, and the two bird species were between these two extremes (Keesing et al. 2009; figure 46). Clearly, the host species on which the tick attempts to feed matters a great deal to tick survival and population dynamics.

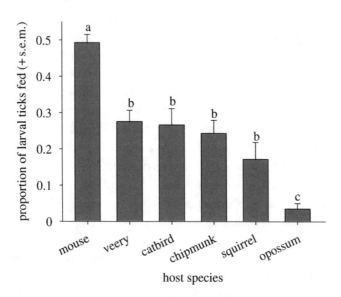

FIGURE 46. The proportions of larval ticks placed on hosts that survived and
fed to repletion. Members of six species were live captured and temporarily taken
to the lab. Each host individual was "treated" with 100 live larval ticks, whose
fates were monitored for the next week. *Source:* Keesing et al. (2009). Reprinted
with permission.

These results demonstrate that some hosts can kill enormous numbers of ticks that encounter them in nature. When we go out into the forest to live trap opossums in August and bring them into the lab for four days, we find that the average opossum feeds 199 larval ticks at any given time. But according to our experimental results, these larvae represent the 3.5% that feed on opossums and survive—the vast majority (96.5%) of larval ticks that encounter an opossum and attempt to feed are apparently consumed during the opossum's grooming. A simple calculation reveals that, during any given week in the summer activity peak for larvae, each opossum must host more than 5,500 larval ticks to produce about 200 that successfully feed, so each opossum kills more than 5,300 larval ticks per week! By this logic, during the larval peak, each mouse encounters approximately 50 larval ticks per week, half of which feed to repletion and become nymphs, with the other half being killed. In an average year we estimate about 25 mice and about one opossum per hectare in our forests; therefore, the mouse population tends to kill about 450 larvae per hectare while the opossum population kills well over 10 times that number. Thus, opossums, and to some extent other nonmouse hosts, serve as ecological traps for larval ticks, concentrating large numbers and then consuming them before they can finish feeding (figure 47). These data provide strong support for the vector-regulation mode of the dilution effect.

The field and lab studies I've just described support the following scenario linking changes in host biodiversity to changes in risk of exposure to Lyme disease. Host communities clearly have different levels of biodiversity. White-footed mice are the only ever-present host, occurring in all communities regardless of the presence of other host species. Mice tend to be most abundant in habitats with few other hosts, particularly predatory hosts. So habitats can be arranged along two interdependent scales—one scale goes from low to high host diversity, and the other goes from high to low abundance of white-footed mice. Low mouse abundance in high-diversity sites appears to be achieved by *host regulation*. If these high-diversity sites with relatively few mice have many other (nonmouse) hosts, we expect tick burdens on mice to be low because the nonmouse hosts intercept ticks that otherwise would have fed on mice (*encounter reduction*). Whenever a high percentage of larval ticks feeds on nonmouse hosts, we expect two consequences: the first is that a lower proportion of the ticks will become infected (because all these other hosts are less efficient reservoirs than are mice); the second is that fewer of the ticks will survive to the nymphal stage (*vector regulation*). Therefore, by three distinct mechanisms, host regulation, encounter reduction, and

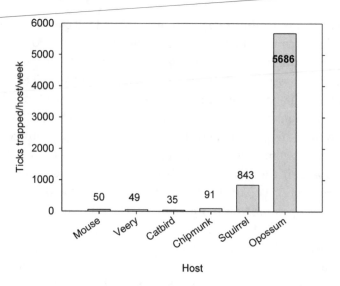

FIGURE 47. Estimated numbers of larval ticks "trapped" and killed by members of six representative host species at sites in Millbrook, New York. The calculations are possible because we have good estimates of the number of larval ticks that feed on an average member of each species, and we have estimated the proportion this number represents out of the total number of ticks that attempt to feed. For more details, see Keesing et al. (2009).

vector regulation, we expect high vertebrate biodiversity to strongly reduce Lyme disease risk.

If we knew where in the landscape vertebrate biodiversity was high and where it was low, we might be able to predict the level of risk and prescribe avoidance or tick control efforts accordingly. Island biogeography theory (MacArthur and Wilson 1967) predicts that smaller habitat "islands" will contain fewer species than will bigger habitat "islands," all else being equal. By virtue of smaller total area, the smaller islands are expected to contain fewer habitat types; any species that rely on the missing habitat types will be lost. In addition, any species that require areas larger than the smaller islands to support viable populations will not be able to persist there. In the midwestern United States, woodlot "islands" in a "sea" of corn and soybean fields do conform to island biogeography theory, with larger woodlots supporting many more species of mammals than do smaller ones (Nupp and Swihart 1998, Rosenblatt et al. 1999). Apparently, these row crops are sufficiently inhospitable to the native mammals that they act as barriers to dispersal in ways similar to oceans surrounding real islands.

If forest fragments in the complex landscapes that characterize Lyme disease zones in the eastern United States act like islands and the areas outside these fragments act like the sea, we might expect diversity to positively correlate with fragment size in these areas. But in these zones some of the habitat types surrounding forest fragments consist of wetlands, abandoned orchards, and old fields, and these seem unlikely to present strong barriers to dispersal. Nevertheless, keeping in mind that island biogeography theory might not apply perfectly to our system, we set out to test the hypothesis that the number of host species would positively correlate with fragment size in our Lyme disease landscapes. Indeed, our aggressive biodiversity surveys in 49 fragments in Dutchess County, New York, revealed such a correlation, also known as *species–area curve* (LoGiudice et al. 2008). Species richness was about 30% higher, on average, in our larger fragments than in our smaller ones (figure 48). There is a fairly high degree of scatter around the species–area curve in figure 48; we think that this is because at least some of the nonforest habitat "seas" allow some species to move through them, and a few species may even regularly occupy them. Such *permeability* of the nonforest habitats would allow some species to be found in forest fragments that, if truly isolated, would be too small to support them.

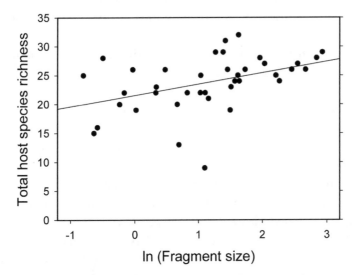

FIGURE 48. The number of mammal and ground-dwelling bird species detected in forest fragments in New York, New Jersey, and Connecticut as a function of fragment size. The significant positive correlation provides an example of a species–area curve and demonstrates that some species drop out of forests as the size of the fragments decrease.

Our observations that the richness of vertebrate species *positively corre-lates* with forest patch size (as one grows, so does the other), and that mouse abundance *negatively correlates* with richness of vertebrate (predator) species (as one increases, the other decreases), suggest where in the landscape risk of exposure to Lyme disease should be highest. We predicted that both the density of nymphal ticks and the proportion of those nymphs that are infected with B. *burgdorferi* would be higher in smaller forest fragments. To test these hypotheses, Brian Allan, Felicia Keesing, and I selected a subset of 14 forest fragments that were as similar as possible in vegetation and in degree of isolation from other suitable habitat for most hosts. We found a significant negative correlation: the larger the forest patch size, the smaller the proportion of nymphs infected with B. *burgdorferi* (figure 49). The infection prevalence values we detected in the smallest fragments are among the highest published values for wild populations of blacklegged ticks, suggesting that the larval tick cohort had little other than highly reservoir-competent white-footed mice on which to feed.

Population density of nymphs also strongly negatively correlated with forest fragment size, although the relationship was not linear. Fragments smaller than about 3 hectares generally supported quite high tick abundances, and tick abundance decreased strongly with increased fragment size, whereas fragments larger than 3 hectares had lower and more constant tick abundances. Multiplying the density of nymphs times the proportion that are infected provides estimates of the density of infected ticks. The pattern for infected nymphs was similar to that for all nymphs, with values on average three to four times higher in smaller than in larger fragments.

Our research has focused largely on the effects of biodiversity, measured by species richness (the number of species in a specific community), on Lyme disease risk. But in some cases the number of species might not be the most appropriate indicator of biodiversity. For example, one could construct two host communities consisting of four species; one of these communities might have white-footed mice, chipmunks, short-tailed shrews, and masked shrews (efficient reservoirs and good hosts), and the other might have raccoons, skunks, opossums, and gray squirrels (poor reservoirs and poor hosts). Despite equal species richness between the two communities, they would produce dramatically different numbers of infected ticks. Such a thought experiment would argue that species *composition*, and not species richness, is the relevant measure of biodiversity for our purposes. I argue above that species richness and species composition are interrelated at least in the community of hosts for blacklegged ticks. As we go from

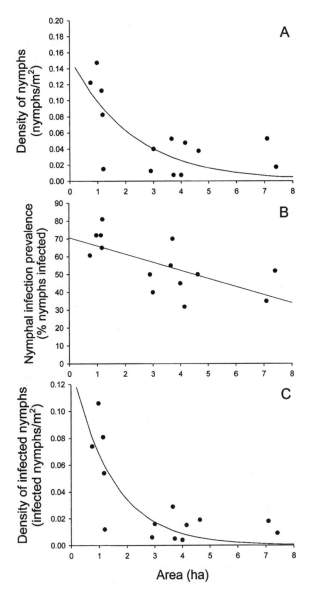

FIGURE 49. The total density of nymphal ticks (top), percentage of nymphs
infected with *B. burgdorferi* (middle), and density of infected nymphs (bottom)
in 14 forest fragments of Dutchess County, New York. *Source*: Allan et al. (2003).
Reprinted with permission.

more species-poor to more species-rich communities, the sequence in
which species are added is at least partly predictable, so we can make
reasonable guesses about which species will occur in more versus less
diverse communities. In essence, we do not find communities consisting only of raccoons, skunks, opossums, and gray squirrels in nature,

so the thought experiment is unfair. Nevertheless, it is worth asking whether our ability to predict Lyme disease risk improves when we have information on species composition compared with data on species richness alone.

Using the proportion of nymphal ticks infected with *B. burgdorferi* (*nymphal infection prevalence*, or NIP) as our measure of Lyme disease risk, my colleagues and I have addressed this question with a combination of field and laboratory studies. NIP for any given cohort of ticks is simply the total number of surviving ticks that got infected during their larval blood meal divided by the total number of surviving larvae that took a blood meal. Breaking this simple equation down further, we know that the total number of larvae that took a blood meal can be estimated by adding up the number of larvae that fed on each host species in the community. If we know the average number of larvae found on an individual of each host species (its *tick burden*) and the total number of individuals (*population density*) of that host species, we can multiply these to produce the total number of ticks fed by each host species in the system. To estimate the number of ticks that got infected during their larval blood meal, we need to multiply the number of larvae that fed on each host species times the proportion of those ticks that become infected (the host's *reservoir competence*). So, to generate an expected value for NIP for any given community, we need estimates for three parameters for each host species—its tick burden, population density, and reservoir competence (Giardina et al. 2000, LoGiudice et al. 2003).

In 2001, Kathleen LoGiudice led our efforts to gather these data for a diverse community of hosts at our field sites in Millbrook, New York. We set out to capture as many members of the vertebrate host community as we possibly could in order to retrieve them to the lab to determine their tick burdens and reservoir competencies. We needed to concentrate this effort in August and early September, because this is the activity period for larval ticks at our sites and elsewhere in the Lyme disease zone of North America. We held captured animals in the laboratory for three to four days, in wire mesh cages suspended over pans of water, because this is how long larval ticks feed before dropping off their hosts. After we counted average body burdens for each host, we maintained each engorged larva in the lab under optimal conditions until it molted into a nymph, and then each nymph was crushed and examined to determine whether it was infected with *B. burgdorferi*, using a direct immunofluorescence assay or polymerase chain reaction. The proportion of nymphs from each host that were infected provided our estimate of host reservoir competence. To estimate host density, either we either used our mark–recapture data, when it was adequate, or we relied on published data from other studies in similar habitats and landscapes.

The data collected in 2001 allowed us to predict that NIP in 2002 would be 0.44 (44% of nymphs infected). To test this prediction, in early summer of 2002, we drag sampled the forest floor with corduroy cloths to collect several hundred nymphs. We determined that NIP was 0.43. The close match between our predicted and observed values of NIP indicated to us that our simple model to predict NIP was valid, that our estimates of the three necessary parameters were accurate, and that we weren't missing an important host in the system. We knew that we hadn't captured all vertebrates that host ticks—some species we failed to catch include red and gray foxes, coyotes, black bears, bobcats, and weasels. However, it seems that these species don't produce sufficient numbers of nymphal ticks to greatly affect the accuracy of our predictions.

Next, we wanted to know how well this approach would serve in predicting NIP in a series of forest fragments in the northeastern United States in which vertebrate diversity varies. We selected 40 fragments in New Jersey, New York, and Connecticut and conducted intensive vertebrate bio-diversity surveys to estimate the abundances of as many host species as we could detect. For some host species, the best we could do in estimating abundance was to categorize them as absent, rare, or common. In these cases, we converted these categories into quantities based on published studies of the species in northeastern forests. Ideally, we would have liked to estimate tick burdens and reservoir competence of each host species in each of the sites, but such a study would be prohibitively expensive. So we relied on the data that we had collected in our Millbrook sites.

Despite clear limitations of our data, we found that the NIP values we measured in each forest fragment highly correlated with the NIP values we predicted in each fragment based on its host species composition (LoGiu-dice et al. 2008; figure 50). Our models tended to overestimate NIP fairly consistently, which suggests that either reservoir competencies or tick bur-dens in Millbrook, or both, are generally higher than for many of the forest fragments. We also used the model to predict how NIP in our Millbrook sites might vary from year to year as the abundance of some of the hosts—particularly mice and chipmunks—varies from year to year. Again, the model produced predictions of NIP that matched the actual values quite well (LoGiudice et al. 2008; figure 51).

We can also use these data to ask whether the specific order in which species disappear as biodiversity declines matters to Lyme disease risk. In

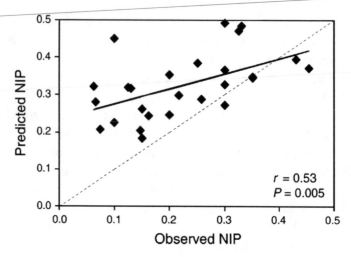

FIGURE 50. Correlation between the nymphal infection prevalence (NIP) predicted by our models from the contributions of each species detected, and the NIP measured in that forest fragment the next year. *Source:* LoGiudice et al. (2008). Reprinted with permission.

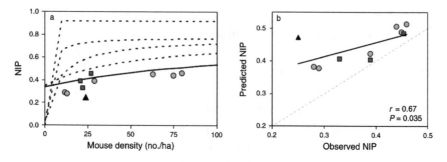

FIGURE 51. The relationship between nymphal infection prevalence (NIP) predicted based on the prior year's density of white-footed mice (left panel, solid line) and measured NIP in the current year (left panel, symbols), and the correlation between annual values of NIP predicted by models and those observed as population densities of mice fluctuated from year to year (right panel). *Source:* LoGiudice et al. (2008). Reprinted with permission.

many cases, we lack strong data to predict which species are most sensitive and which are least sensitive to the forces that erode biodiversity. Destruction and fragmentation of habitat is the most potent cause of biodiversity loss worldwide (Primack 2006), and this is likely true of the North American forests that are affected by Lyme disease. Several plausible models, or rules of thumb, might describe the sequence of species loss under habitat loss/fragmentation. These include a body size rule, whereby larger species are lost first; a home range rule, in which more widely ranging species are lost first; and a trophic level rule, whereby the more carnivorous species are the first to go. In addition to these theoretically plausible models, data exist from the midwestern U.S. forest fragments described above that might apply to the landscapes of the Lyme disease zone. As a contrast to these orderly rules of "community disassembly," one might include a null model whereby the sequence of species loss is entirely random (that is, there are no rules). Because we know the effects that each host species has on NIP, we can use computer simulations to ask whether these different rules (including the null model) give rise to different predictions about how NIP will change as biodiversity is lost.

Such simulations show, in fact, that the rules governing the sequence of species loss in nature are profoundly important. Under the null model that species are lost in an entirely random sequence, NIP declines dramatically with biodiversity loss (figure 52), a result that is directly contradicted by our data (Ostfeld and LoGiudice 2003, LoGiudice et al. 2008). If we simply assume that white-footed mice are present everywhere

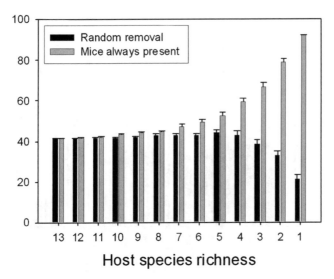

Host species richness

FIGURE 52. Results of a simulation model in which nymphal infection prevalence (NIP) changes as species richness in the host community varies. Two community disassembly rules are represented: the null model, in which species are removed in random sequence, and the quasi-null rule, in which mice are assumed to be present in all communities and all other species are removed in random sequence. Bars represent means with standard errors from 100 simulations at each level of species richness. For more details, see Ostfeld and LoGiudice (2003). *Source:* Ostfeld et al. (2006b). Reprinted with permission.

(supported by our data), and otherwise assume that species are lost in random order, we find the exact opposite result, that NIP increases dramatically with biodiversity loss (figure 52). Application of the more nuanced rules of thumb (body size, home range size, and trophic level) shows strong increases in NIP with biodiversity loss, but the shapes of the curves vary somewhat (figure 53). This exercise suggests that knowing which species are most and least sensitive to habitat loss and fragmentation will increase our ability to predict the consequences for human risk of Lyme disease.

The roles that different host species play in affecting Lyme disease risk depend not only on how many ticks they feed and infect, but also on how many ticks they kill. Experiments described above (see figure 46) show how dramatically the various vertebrate hosts differ in their likelihood of killing larval blacklegged ticks that try to feed on them. Although these data are available for only six of our host species, we can use these six species to predict the effects of changes in biodiversity on the *density of infected nymphs* (DIN), in addition to NIP. What we wish to ask here is

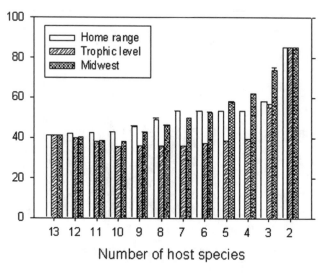

FIGURE 53. Results of a simulation model in which nymphal infection prevalence (NIP) changes under three nonrandom disassembly rules: the body size/home range size rule, in which species with larger bodies/home ranges are lost first; the trophic level rule, in which the most carnivorous species are lost first; and the "Midwest rule," in which species are lost in roughly the order observed in fragmented landscapes in the midwestern United States. For more details, see Ostfeld and LoGiudice (2003). *Source:* Ostfeld et al. (2006b). Reprinted with permission.

how many infected nymphs we expect to find in a given community. We can address this question only because we have collected detailed information on each species' average body burden, population density, reservoir competence, and *host quality*, measured by tick survival rates.

Again, we start with a maximally species-rich community and select species for removal, in a sequence that is supported by data from previous studies. To make these models more realistic, we must try to account for the fates of the larval ticks that would have fed on a host species had that host been present. In other words, when modeling species removals from a host community, one can assume that all of the ticks that would have fed on the host (if it were present) also disappear, or that all of them find a host of another species, or that some percentage disappears and the rest find an alternate host. To cover this range of possibilities, we allowed the "redistribution rate" of the ticks from removed hosts to vary from zero to 100%. For these models, we removed veeries first, because this bird prefers forest interiors and tends not to occupy edges or small fragments. Next, we removed opossums because they are relatively large-bodied and require large home ranges. The rest of the sequence was gray squirrels, followed by chipmunks, and then gray catbirds, reflecting published data by our group and others (LoGiudice et al. 2008, Rosenblatt et al. 1999).

Although removal of veeries had only a modest effect on Lyme disease risk, measured by DIN, as additional host species were removed DIN rose substantially (figure 54). Species removals increased Lyme disease risk most strongly when a large percentage of larval ticks were redistributed onto other hosts, but even when only 10–15% of larval ticks were redistributed, species removals still resulted in increased risk. This exercise tells us two things. First, the loss of biodiversity increases Lyme disease risk, whether that risk is measured by NIP or by DIN. Second, in order to understand the size of the effect, we must learn more about how ticks respond to changes in the relative or absolute abundance of different host species. Our studies show that having more chipmunks in the host community translates directly into fewer ticks on mice, which suggests that the distribution of ticks across the host community is highly sensitive to the composition of that community. This would mean that ticks in a community that loses a host are likely to redistribute themselves among the remaining hosts to a large degree. Confirming this expectation, though, awaits further study.

Our simulation modeling also revealed that the effects of losing any given species from a host community might differ depending on which other species remain in the community. We found, for instance, that when

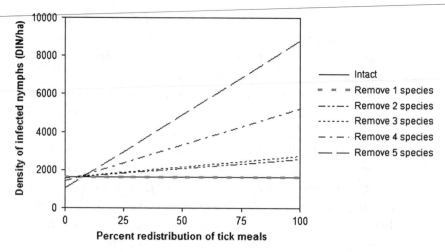

FIGURE 54. The density of infected nymphal ticks (DIN) per hectare as host species were removed sequentially from our model (Keesing et al. 2009), when 0–100% of the ticks that would have fed on the missing hosts were redistributed among remaining hosts. Species were removed from the model in an order determined by empirical observations of the sequence of species loss in fragmented forest habitats. In habitats with two or more species lost, DIN was higher if ticks were redistributed on remaining hosts, and greater rates of redistribution resulted in higher values of DIN. Updated from Keesing et al. (2009).

shrews or chipmunks are lost from a low-diversity community, the result is likely to be an increase in NIP, but when they are lost from a high-diversity community, the result is a strong decrease in NIP (figure 55). In the parlance of community ecology, the functional roles played by species are not constant but rather depend on, or are *contingent* upon, certain ecological conditions, in this case the composition of the remaining community (Ostfeld and LoGiudice 2003, Ostfeld et al. 2006b).

One biomedical example of ecological contingencies is the effect of antibiotics on bacterial communities in human guts. *Clostridium difficile* is a bacterial member of our gut flora, and in most people it causes no detectable health problems. However, when some people take antibiotics for bacterial infections such as urinary tract or upper respiratory infections, the existing *C. difficile* populations in their guts can increase dramatically in abundance and secrete toxins that cause severe stomach pain, diarrhea, and in up to 15% of cases, death (Dixon and Menezes 2009) Apparently, *C. difficile* normally is benign in the human intestines because its abundance and toxic secretions are strongly regulated by other naturally occurring bacteria. But when antibiotic use destroys some of these other gut bacteria, *C. difficile* changes its functional role to that of a killer (Lawley et al. 2009). When species'

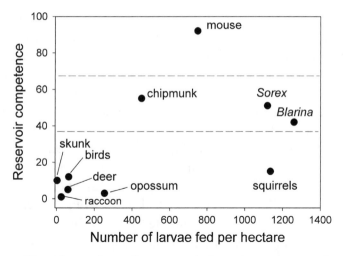

FIGURE 55. Different effects of losing a species from a host community, based on which species remain. Each host species in the graph is located in "phase space," defined as the combination of reservoir competence, as measured in the field (and number of larvae fed by that host species per hectare. The *reservoir competence* axis indicates whether that species increases or decreases total nymphal infection prevalence (NIP), and the *number of larvae fed* axis indicates how large or small an effect that species has on total NIP. In a fully intact community at our field sites in Millbrook, New York, NIP values range between 35% and 40% (lower dashed line), whereas in species-poor communities, NIP is much higher (upper dashed line; see Allan et al. 2003). In a species-poor community, with high NIP, loss of such species as shrews (*Sorex* and *Blarina* species) and chipmunks would increase NIP even further. But in a species-rich community, with lower NIP, loss of these same species would reduce NIP even further. *Source:* Ostfeld et al. (2006b). Reprinted with permission.

functional roles change in magnitude and even in direction (for example, from positive or neutral to negative), our ability to predict the consequences of ecological change can be diminished. However, because such contingencies seem to pervade ecological systems (including human bodies), it is critical for ecologists and managers of those systems to recognize and account for this context dependence. The importance of such ecological contingencies in vector-borne diseases has only begun to be explored.

Chapter 2 describes how medical entomologists and epidemiologists aggressively sought *the* critical tick host and *the* critical pathogen reservoir in the early years after the emergence of Lyme disease. Despite clear early evidence that several or even many vertebrate species were involved in maintaining tick populations, and that these hosts differed strongly in their probability of infecting ticks, researchers homed in on deer as the maintenance host and mice as the reservoir host. Chapters 3 and 4 show how inadequately such a two-host model represents the Lyme disease system. Only after more than 20 years of field and laboratory studies on tick–host interactions did researchers begin to take seriously the fact that blacklegged tick and *B. burgdorferi* populations are affected profoundly by many different hosts.

It is interesting to speculate about how our knowledge would differ today had researchers accepted from the start the broad distribution of ticks across dozens of host species, each of which has unique effects on tick abundance and infection. What if we had started with a model in which the main risk factor, the density of infected nymphs (DIN), was recognized to be the product of three basic parameters specific to each host—how many larval ticks it feeds (body burden per host times host density), how many of those larval ticks get infected (reservoir competence), and how many larval ticks it kills (host "quality"), summed over the host community? I'd hazard a guess that we would have developed more effective, community-based measures for controlling numbers of infected ticks at a much earlier stage and prevented many cases of Lyme disease. Lyme disease would also seem to provide an excellent model for approaching other emerging zoonotic diseases, which I discuss in chapter 9.

Human Dimensions of Lyme Disease Risk and Incidence

Although we need to understand what causes variations in tick abundance and infection prevalence in order to understand variations in Lyme disease risk, two recent studies highlight the limitations of understanding ecological risk to predict patterns of exposure in people. Brownstein and colleagues (2005) found that, although tick density and infection prevalence were higher in Connecticut sites where forest cover was highly fragmented, the incidence rates of Lyme disease in people showed the opposite pattern—lowest in the most highly fragmented sites. In another study in Maryland, Jackson and colleagues (2006a) found that high rates of Lyme disease in humans were associated with portions of the landscape containing edges between forest and herbaceous plant communities (for example, lawns, golf courses, old fields). However, our studies in New York (Horobik et al. 2006) clearly indicate that edges themselves are not risky habitat types—they have dramatically fewer ticks than adjacent forests (figure 56). A major implication of these studies is that entomological/ecological risk,

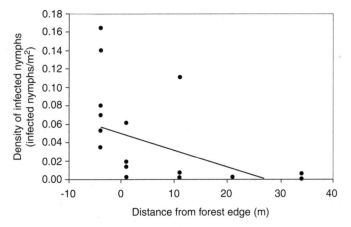

FIGURE 56. Density of infected nymphal blacklegged ticks by distance from the edges of forests and grassy fields, at the Cary Institute in Millbrook, New York. Zero represents the edge itself; negative numbers represent samples taken in forests, and positive numbers represent samples taken in the fields at various distances from the forest edge. *Source:* Horobik et al. (2006). Reprinted with permission.

while important, might poorly predict epidemiological patterns. I suspect that in some cases human behaviors, and the knowledge and attitudes from which they arise, are responsible for the lack of agreement between ecological risk and actual cases of Lyme disease. For example, people may have low rates of contracting Lyme disease in highly fragmented sites because they don't often use these "forested" components of urban landscapes, even though infected ticks abound there. Similarly, forest–field edges might be risky "habitats" because people use them more frequently, rather than because abundance of infected ticks is particularly high.

Use of habitats is not the only variable affecting exposure to Lyme disease risk; humans also can protect themselves in several ways. Although a vaccine for Lyme disease was available for several years in the late 1990s, it is no longer produced, and new vaccine development appears years away. Consequently, avoiding bites by infected ticks and quickly removing embedded ticks are the only direct preventive measures available. Avoidance strategies include avoiding tick habitat (primarily forests) during early summer (nymphal activity peak), wearing protective clothing, using insect repellents, adopting landscaping practices that discourage tick entry or survival, and daily grooming to inspect for and remove ticks. At the landscape level, long-term strategies to reduce Lyme incidence might include more clustered residential and commercial development that leads to less forest fragmentation.

The few studies that have examined behavioral correlates of Lyme disease have identified several associations between human behaviors and Lyme disease risk, including daily activities like gardening (Orloski et al. 1998, Armstrong et al. 2001, Poland 2001), level of personal protection (Fish 1995, Poland 2001), and residential proximity to forested areas (Cromley et al. 1998). This suggests that a combination of information about ticks, risk perception, and behaviors—both risk enhancing and risk reducing—are important factors in exposure to Lyme disease and subsequent infection. In this context, it's interesting to speculate about the potential for a feedback loop from human management of forested landscapes, to changes in entomological risk of Lyme disease (DIN or NIP), to knowledge that biodiversity loss from certain types of forest destruction and fragmentation increases risk, to changes in behaviors that affect forest destruction (figure 57). There is little doubt that the fragmentation of

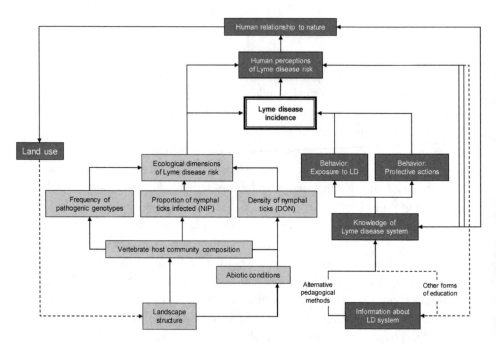

FIGURE 57. Conceptual model of linkages in the Lyme disease system. Lyme disease incidence is a function of both ecological dimensions of risk (light shading) and human dimensions of risk (dark shading), including knowledge and behaviors. Perceptions of risk, and the consequences of this perception, might produce feedbacks that influence both ecological dynamics and human behavior. Solid arrows represent interactions that have been addressed at least partially by empirical research; dashed arrows are for future study. Diagram drawn by F. Keesing.

forests that accompanies certain types of residential and industrial development increases ecological risk to users of the remaining forest. Knowledge of this effect of development might cause some people to avoid exposure to infected ticks or to control tick populations in risky areas. But it could also change attitudes about the types of development most likely to increase risk, resulting in alternative types of development (or none at all) that don't increase risk. To my knowledge, researchers have not yet approached this question.

9

Embracing Complexity

Ecosystem Functioning

WITHOUT A DOUBT, ONE OF THE HOTTEST ISSUES IN ECOLOGY OVER the past decade is the relationship between biodiversity and ecosystem function. Does biodiversity matter to the way that ecosystems perform? Naturalists have known since antiquity that ecological communities differ dramatically in their biodiversity. Tropical rain forests and coral reefs are the quintessential examples of highly diverse biomes, whereas tundras and salt marshes are much less diverse. Even ecosystems sitting side by side can differ strongly—think of a cornfield next to a tall-grass prairie, or a rocky intertidal zone next to a sandy one. And the same piece of real estate can be transformed from high to low diversity or vice versa. For instance, conversion of tropical forest to cattle pasture destroys most of its biodiversity, whereas natural succession of sand dune to grassland and ultimately forest is accompanied by a major rise in biodiversity. Ecologists have been asking whether it matters that biodiversity is gained or lost in an ecosystem, and if so, how.

Biodiversity everywhere on the planet is being massively destroyed at a rate that is unprecedented even considering the most precipitous mass extinctions in Earth's history, such as that of the dinosaurs at the end of the Cretaceous Period. For example, 2,000 species of Pacific Island birds have gone extinct since human colonization of those islands in the past few centuries; 120 species of amphibians have gone extinct since 1980, and 32% of those that remain are considered threatened; at current rates of extinction, up to 50% of all mammal species will disappear within the next 200 years (Ceballos and Ehrlich 2002). All of these statistics refer to permanent, irrevocable extinctions of entire species. But extinctions and near-extinctions of populations (groups of organisms of the same species living in the same place at the same time) are undoubtedly far more frequent and far less documented than are species extinctions.

The vast majority of these extinctions are caused or accelerated by a wide variety of human activities. The principle human activity that causes local or global extinction is habitat destruction (Turner et al. 2007, Brook et al. 2008). Habitat destruction itself is caused by exploitation of natural resources (such as mining, logging, damming) and the replacement of native habitat by human constructs (for example, urban and suburban sprawl, agricultural fields). In all these cases, the economic well-being of people that benefit, directly or indirectly, from exploitation of resources or habitat conversion is the main driving force. Biodiversity loss is considered by some to be either unimportant or perhaps an unfortunate yet necessary casualty of economic growth and human progress. The benefits of activities that result in biodiversity loss are often quite apparent, immediate, and measurable in dollars or other currency—higher beef production, hydroelectric power, new suburban developments. In contrast, the costs of the resulting biodiversity loss are often cryptic, delayed, and not easily measured by standard units. As a consequence, those who advocate for activities that destroy biodiversity are able to support their projects with benefits that appear to vastly outweigh costs.

So, what *are* the costs of losing biodiversity, or conversely, what are the benefits of preserving biodiversity? These can be divided, imperfectly, into utilitarian and nonutilitarian categories. The *nonutilitarian benefits* of preserving biodiversity are driven by esthetically, ethically, and morally derived values placed on the perpetuation and promotion of diverse forms of life. Advocates of this view argue that we humans have an ethical obligation to preserve the variety of life forms with which we share the planet, and that projects that would destroy important components of biodiversity should be altered or prevented to reduce the damage. In most situations, the promoters of development projects that would cause substantial biodiversity loss have no trouble undermining such contrarian, nonutilitarian arguments, because the project's tangible economic benefits are so obvious. Mega-dams, mountaintop removals for coal mining, and offshore oil drilling come to mind as clear examples of projects that proceed despite causing immense destruction of biodiversity. Esthetic and moral concerns tend not to get in the way. On the other hand, if the loss of biodiversity were to adversely affect more tangible, utilitarian aspects of human well-being, then the cost–benefit calculations could change profoundly. For example, if the conversion of tropical forest to pasture destroyed an ecotourism industry that depended on biodiversity, or if offshore drilling for oil imperiled the marine biodiversity that supports a lucrative fishery, then such development projects are more likely to be altered or scrapped.

In recent years ecologists have aggressively sought to identify *utilitarian functions* that are served by high biodiversity and compromised when biodiversity is lost. In general, ecologists have focused on a rather limited subset of possible utilitarian functions of biodiversity, for example, rates of nutrient cycling, primary production, and resistance to disturbances such as drought (Naeem et al. 2009). Both carefully designed experiments and correlational or comparative studies repeatedly support the hypothesis that these ecosystem functions are performed more efficiently in more diverse than in less diverse communities (Naeem et al. 2009). One might think that demonstrating tangible benefits of biodiversity would help inform debates over the costs and benefits of development projects that might destroy biodiversity. Ironically, it appears that non-ecologists are not aware of or not impressed by the enhanced nutrient cycling and primary production achieved in highly diverse communities. For instance, a 2007 European Union survey showed that considerably more respondents consider moral reasons stronger than utilitarian reasons for protecting biodiversity (European Commission 2007). In a 2002 survey in the United States (Biodiversity Project 2002), utilitarian and economic functions of biodiversity, with the exception of human health, are not even mentioned.

But, what if the loss of biodiversity made you sick? What if it made you and your family more likely to be exposed to infectious diseases, or made the food and fiber crops you depend on more likely to be attacked by pathogens? Chapter 8 presents evidence that the loss of vertebrate biodiversity from landscapes in the northeastern United States increases the abundance and infection prevalence of blacklegged ticks, which directly increases risk of human exposure to Lyme disease. I describe how the expectation that biodiversity loss will increase disease risk arises from two separate philosophical approaches to scientific knowing—a deductive one, in which epidemiological theory is used to derive generalized expectations, and an inductive one, in which the compilation of field and laboratory information on a given disease system (Lyme disease) generates specific predictions that might then be generalized to other systems.

The purpose of this chapter is to ask whether biodiversity loss increases risk in other infectious diseases of humans and other organisms. If such an effect is common, then the impact of biodiversity loss on the health of humans, wildlife, domestic stock, and important plants and microbes must be incorporated into permitting, regulating, and managing potentially destructive development projects. To address this question I review some recent case studies of the impact of changes in biodiversity on disease dynamics. I follow this review with a speculative discussion of why the loss of biodiversity appears to usually increase disease transmission rather than reduce it. Last, I argue that the protection of human, wildlife, other animal, and plant health should be viewed as an ecosystem function alongside the more traditionally studied functions like primary production and nutrient cycling.

Hantavirus Pulmonary Syndrome

The hantaviruses (family Bunyaviridae) cause such severe, untreatable illnesses that they are included by the Centers for Disease Control and Prevention as Category C bioterrorism agents/diseases, defined as, "emerging pathogens that could be engineered for mass dissemination in the future because of availability, ease of production and dissemination, and potential for high morbidity and mortality rates and major health impact (CDC 2010) . When hantaviruses invade human bodies, they damage tissues that line the capillaries, causing massive leakage of fluids into surrounding tissues. Depending on which tissues are affected, hantavirus infections can cause severe hemorrhaging, kidney malfunction, or drowning when air spaces in the lung fill with fluid. Hantaviruses as a group were first discovered in the early 1950s when thousands of Korean War soldiers fell ill with severe kidney disease and hemorrhagic fever. For decades the hantaviruses were thought to be limited to portions of Asia and Europe.

But in 1993, researchers at the U.S. Centers for Disease Control and Prevention who were pursuing a highly lethal pulmonary (lung) illness that erupted in the southwestern United States discovered a new North American hantavirus. By tradition, discoverers of previously undescribed pathogenic viruses name them after the location where they first emerge. So the newly described North American hantavirus, which causes hantavirus pulmonary syndrome, was named Four Corners hantavirus after the region where the states of New Mexico, Utah, Colorado, and Arizona meet. Anticipating bad publicity, authorities in the Four Corners area pressured virologists to name it something else, but when virologists tried to use more local geographic names for the virus, the same thing happened, over and over, until finally they chose to use the name Sin Nombre ("no name") virus.

Since that time, several other species of hantaviruses that cause lung or heart and lung disease have been discovered in the Americas, especially in Patagonia (Argentina, Brazil, and Chile) and Panama. Fatality rates for those infected with these viruses are often between 20% and 50% (Yates et al. 2002). Each species of hantavirus tends to be associated with a particular species of rodent that acts as a reservoir, although the species-to-species association is not perfect. For example, Sin Nombre hantavirus is largely limited to deer mice (*Peromyscus maniculatus*) but also can persist in other, related rodents. Whether infections in non-deer-mouse hosts result from *spillover* (occasional transmission events from deer mice that do not result in amplification within the "accidental" host) or represent the ability of the virus to proliferate in these other hosts (that is, to use them as a reservoir) is not known. Hantaviruses apparently are transmitted from rodent to rodent during fights or other close encounters when infected individuals bite, scratch, or lick uninfected individuals (Yates et al. 2002). Human exposure to hantavirus occurs when we inhale aerosols containing bits of rodent urine, feces, or saliva with virus particles. Because these particles degrade rapidly, when rodent excreta is subjected to sunlight and warm temperatures, hantaviruses don't persist for more than a few days.

Rodent reservoirs tend to shed virus particles most abundantly in the first days and weeks after exposure. As soon as they enter a susceptible host, viruses tend to invade tissues and reproduce, or *replicate*, rapidly, reaching high concentrations in mucus membranes, the bladder, and the intestines before the host is able to mount an effective immune response. Within a few weeks, antibody production induced by the infection dramatically reduces shedding rates, and the immunity that is produced prevents the animal from becoming reinfected by future exposures (Yates et al. 2002). Thus, researchers have focused on identifying the factors that cause widespread transmission of new infections within reservoir populations. Several studies have shown that human incidence of hantavirus disease is highest when populations of infected reservoir hosts are densest in and around human dwellings (Kuenzi et al. 2001, Yates et al. 2002). Other studies suggest that the proportion of reservoir hosts currently infected or the rate of transmission events in the reservoir population is the best predictor of human risk (Yates et al. 2002, Sauvage et al. 2007).

So, how might biodiversity affect risk of human exposure to hantavirus? As described in chapter 8, surveillance studies that examine natural

communities of small mammals to identify the reservoir for specific hantaviruses tend to find a single reservoir species for each hantavirus (Yates
et al. 2002). The list of reservoir hosts for the various hantaviruses (Yates
et al. 2002, their figure 3) includes the Norway rat (*Rattus norvegicus*), the
meadow vole (*Microtus pennsylvanicus*), the deer mouse (*Peromyscus maniculatus*), the white-footed mouse (*P. leucopus*), the hispid cotton rat (*Sig-
modon hispidus*), the rice rat (*Oryzomys palustris*), and the small vesper
mouse (*Calomys laucha*). Each of these species is well known to be highly
abundant, widespread, resilient, and a habitat generalist. Most or all of
these species respond favorably to many types of habitat disturbance (for
example, urbanization, deforestation, agriculture). Based on the discussion of the dilution effect in chapter 8, therefore, we might expect that high
biodiversity could reduce exposure risk in at least two ways. First, if high
biodiversity in the vertebrate community reduces the abundance of the
reservoir host, then risk of human exposure is likely to decline with
increases in biodiversity according to the *host regulation* mechanism.
Second, if high vertebrate biodiversity reduces rates of encounter between
infectious and susceptible reservoir hosts, then risk of exposure will decline
with increases in biodiversity according to the *encounter reduction* mechanism. Studies in North America and Panama find strong support for a
dilution effect that seems to be produced by both these mechanisms.

The first assessment of a dilution effect in hantavirus disease was an
analysis by Ostfeld and Keesing (2000a) of a study by Mills and colleagues
(1998), who surveyed deer mice from nine different U.S. national parks for
infection prevalence (*seroprevalence*), and also presented data on the
number of small mammal species they trapped at those locations. Ostfeld
and Keesing hypothesized that the existence of a dilution effect would be
supported if the average proportion of deer mice infected was lower in
communities with more small mammal species. Although the data did
appear to support their hypothesis—the relationship between small
mammal biodiversity and hantavirus infection prevalence in deer mice did
appear to be negative—the correlation was not statistically significant
(Ostfeld and Keesing 2000a). A follow-up study by Calisher and colleagues
(2002) measured small mammal biodiversity and hantavirus prevalence at
three sites in western Colorado. At one of the sites, only two small mammal
species were present, and seroprevalence in deer mice was 13%. At a second site, four species occurred and seroprevalence was 9%. At the third
site, 19 species were captured and seroprevalence was 2%. Although it is
difficult to statistically analyze a correlation based on three sites, the data
appear consistent with the dilution effect.

A more recent study by Dizney and Ruedas (2009) assessed the relationship between mammalian biodiversity and the seroprevalence of Sin Nombre hantavirus in deer mouse reservoirs at five sites in and around Portland, Oregon. The five sites were selected to represent a broad range of mammal biodiversity. Extensive trapping for mammals of all sizes was conducted over three years, resulting in the capture of more than 5,000 individuals from 21 species. The results were dramatic. Seroprevalence in deer mice was low (about 2%) in all sites that had moderate to high mammal biodiversity but was seven times as high, about 14%, in the site with the lowest biodiversity (figure 58). The data fit the model extraordinarily well (an exponential decay curve explained >99% of the variation in the data), which strongly supports the dilution effect.

Dizney and Ruedas (2009) did not find, however, that the hantavirus infection prevalence was higher in denser mouse populations, or that mouse density was lower in more diverse communities. Consequently, their data do not support the host regulation mechanism. Instead, they interpret their results as supporting the encounter reduction mechanism of the dilution effect (Keesing et al. 2006). Many of the species that occurred in the high-diversity sites were predators on deer mice, and the presence of predators is known to reduce movement rates and other activity levels of small mammal prey (Dizney and Ruedas 2009). Perhaps an abundance of diverse predators curtails encounters between individual deer mice, resulting in far fewer transmissions of hantavirus (Dizney and Ruedas 2009). This study suggests that a threshold level of mammalian biodiversity is

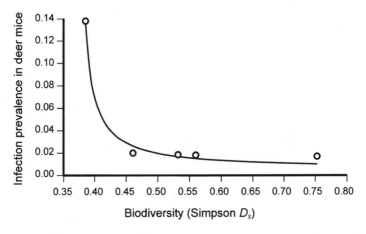

FIGURE 58. Prevalence of Sin Nombre hantavirus infection in populations of deer mice *(Peromyscus maniculatus)* as a function of mammal species diversity at sites in Oregon. *Source:* Dizney and Ruedas (2009). Reprinted with permission.

necessary to suppress hantavirus transmission, and that below this threshold risk of human exposure could be quite high. Another recent study of North American hantavirus ecology suggested that a high diversity of species that compete with deer mice can reduce population density either through mortality or emigration, thereby reducing prevalence of Sin Nombre virus infection (Clay et al. 2009).

A hantavirus called Puumala virus has been causing severe kidney disease in residents of northern Europe for decades. The reservoir for this virus is a small forest rodent called the bank vole (*Myodes glareolus*). In some forests, bank voles are much more common than the other common forest-floor rodent, the wood mouse (*Apodemus sylvaticus*), whereas in other localities wood mice are more common. A recent study conducted in Belgium found that infection prevalence in bank voles (which represented human risk) was significantly higher in forests where bank voles were common and wood mice were scarce, and lower in forests where bank voles and wood mice were equally common (Tersago et al. 2008). Although the total number of species (two) remained the same, when both species were well represented (that is, species evenness was high), disease transmission was low.

In the Azuero Peninsula of southern Panama, an outbreak of hantavirus pulmonary syndrome occurred in late 1999 and 2000, killing more than one out of every five people who were exposed. A newly recognized hantavirus, named Choclo virus, was implicated as the agent of human illness, and a second, previously undescribed hantavirus, Calabazo virus, was also detected in the region. The reservoir for Choclo virus was determined to be the pigmy rice rat, *Oligoryzomys fulvescens*, and the reservoir for Calabazo virus was identified as the cane mouse, *Zygodontomys brevicauda*. Both of these species are highly resilient rodents that increase in numbers when habitats are disturbed or otherwise altered by human activities (for example, conversion of forest to pasture and agriculture) (Ruedas et al. 2004). In undisturbed ecosystems of the Azuero Peninsula, many other small mammal species occur, but most of these species become scarce or absent altogether when these habitats are converted to pasture, row crops, or human habitations.

During the waning period of the outbreak of hantavirus pulmonary syndrome, Ruedas and colleagues (2004) established research sites at 12 locations where hantavirus pulmonary syndrome had been confirmed in at least one human patient and at one additional site where no disease had been detected. Using live-trapping methods, the group measured small mammal biodiversity and the proportion of reservoir hosts (*O. fulvescens* and *Z. brevicauda*) that were infected with and producing antibodies to the hantaviruses. They found that the one undisturbed site with no cases of hantavirus disease had significantly higher small mammal biodiversity than did any of the disturbed sites with hantavirus pulmonary syndrome. This result is consistent with the dilution effect, but the study provided no information on possible mechanism.

A few years later, Gerardo Suzan and colleagues (2009) undertook a rigorous experimental study in the Azuero Peninsula to assess whether the dilution effect occurs in this disease and, if so, by what mechanisms. Suzan established 24 sites in forest fragments in and around the zone that had been afflicted by hantavirus pulmonary syndrome. The sites were divided into 16 experimental and eight control sites, assuring that the two categories did not differ in habitat, elevation, and landscape context. The experimental design was simple but unprecedented. The researchers undertook regular, monthly live trapping of all small mammals on all sites. On the experimental sites, all trapped individuals from nonreservoir species were permanently removed, whereas all the pigmy rice rats and cane mice were marked and released according to standard procedures. On the control sites, all individuals from all species, nonreservoirs and the two reservoir species alike, were simply marked and released.

The removal of nonreservoir species from the experimental sites (that is, the experimental reduction of biodiversity) had a dramatic effect on the abundance of the two reservoir species. In the control sites where no species were removed, abundance of pigmy rice rats and cane mice declined steadily throughout the study period, presumably as a result of seasonal decline in reproduction (Suzan et al. 2009; figure 59). But when nonreservoirs were removed, this decline was largely alleviated, with the result that abundance of reservoirs was significantly higher (figure 59). The higher reservoir density in experimental sites suggests that the nonreservoirs that were removed compete with, or prey on, the reservoirs. Perhaps even more striking than the effect of nonreservoir removal on the *abundance* of reservoirs was the effect on the *proportion of reservoirs infected with hantavirus.* In control sites, the proportion of reservoirs testing positive for hantavirus was between 8% and 12%. However, where nonreservoirs were removed, seroprevalence in the two reservoirs increased from 15% to 35%, ultimately reaching levels more than three times as high on experimental sites as on the control sites (figure 60).

The experimental reduction in small mammal biodiversity in Panama supports two distinct mechanisms of the dilution effect. The increase in reservoir abundance when biodiversity was reduced supports the host

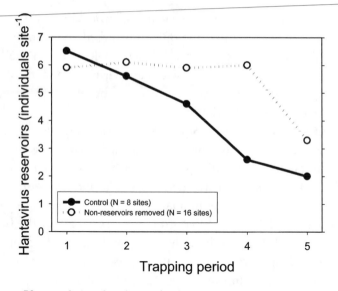

FIGURE 59. Population abundance of rodent reservoirs for hantaviruses in the Azuero Peninsula, Panama, where nonreservoir species were removed during monthly live trapping (experimental sites) and where no species were removed (controls). Data from Suzan et al. (2009).

regulation mechanism. And because the proportion of reservoirs infected was significantly higher when nonreservoirs were removed, it seems that biodiversity loss also increased encounter rates between hosts, boosting transmission events. Although much more work remains to understand mechanisms, the data support a strong protective effect of high small mammal diversity on key elements of human risk of exposure to hantaviruses in North America, Central America, and Europe.

West Nile Virus Disease

West Nile virus is a flavivirus (relative of yellow fever virus) that can cause serious disease in a wide range of vertebrate hosts, including humans. Although some human infections produce only mild flulike symptoms or no noticeable symptoms at all, other West Nile virus infections can cause inflammation of the brain and spinal cord and even death in 3% to 15% of cases (CDC 2009). The disease was first discovered in the West Nile district of Uganda in 1937, and later outbreaks occurred in central and northern Africa, Israel, eastern and southern Europe, and Russia. In 1999, the virus suddenly appeared in New York City, probably having been introduced by

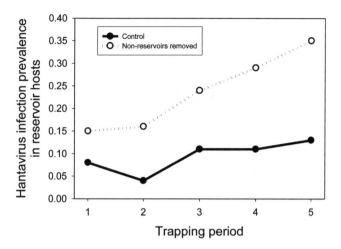

FIGURE 60. Prevalence of hantavirus infection of rodent reservoirs in the Azuero Peninsula, Panama, where nonreservoir species were removed during monthly live trapping (experimental sites) and where no species were removed (controls). Data from Suzan et al. (2009).

tourists who had been exposed while visiting Israel (Despommier 2001). By the time the virus had made itself known by sickening dozens of people and killing hundreds of crows and other birds, it was already entrenched in North America and rapidly spreading. In four short years West Nile virus had spread all the way to California and had penetrated all 48 contiguous states.

West Nile virus replicates within the bodies of a number of bird species. Several of these species tend to produce high concentrations of virus particles in their blood (*viremias*) that persist for several days before their immune systems are able to clear the infection. Some other species produce high viremias but die quickly from disease. Yet others are more resistant to infection, producing only modest viremias with or without illness. West Nile virus is transmitted among hosts almost exclusively by the bite of certain species of mosquito (rare cases of direct host-to-host transmission have been documented in the lab, but their frequency in nature is unknown). The most important vectors in North America are in the mosquito genus *Culex*. Mosquitoes that bite highly viremic hosts are likely to become infected and able to transmit a substantial dose of virus to other hosts during later blood meals. The higher the concentration of virus in host blood and the longer the host maintains that concentration, the greater the *reservoir competence* of the host. Laboratory studies of birds, mammals, and some reptiles have shown that a handful of bird species are the most competent reservoirs for West Nile virus. These include the blue jay, common grackle, American crow, American robin, house finch, and house sparrow (Komar et al. 2003, 2005). Most other birds, including both songbirds (*passerines*) and nonpasserines, as well as mammals and reptiles do not sufficiently amplify virus to act as competent reservoirs.

Perusal of this list of the most competent West Nile virus reservoirs immediately suggests a common thread—all these birds tend to be most abundant in human-dominated landscapes, including cities and suburbs, where avian diversity is generally low. They are considerably less common or even absent in more natural landscapes, including intact forests, where avian diversity is high (Allan et al. 2009). Imagine two groups of adult female mosquitoes searching for blood meals from a community of vertebrate hosts. One group exists within a disturbed ecosystem dominated by crows, finches, sparrows, and robins, and the other forages in an intact forest ecosystem with few of these birds and many other species with low reservoir competence. It stands to reason that the first group of mosquitoes would have higher infection prevalence, and that any people in the area would therefore be at greater risk of exposure to West Nile virus. Because of the correlation between reservoir competence and resilience to human disturbance, one might expect the dilution effect to operate in the West Nile virus system.

Vanessa Ezenwa and colleagues were the first to ask whether the dilution effect occurs for this pathogen. Based on the observation that nonpasserine birds are almost always poor West Nile virus reservoirs, Ezenwa and colleagues (2006) hypothesized that virus infection rates in both mosquitoes and people would be lower in areas with greater numbers of nonpasserine species. To test the hypotheses, this group collected mosquitoes, determined how many were infected with the virus, and estimated the number of bird species, in six sites within St. Tammany Parish, in eastern Louisiana. They found that mosquito infection prevalence strongly, negatively correlated with the diversity (species richness) of nonpasserine birds, supporting the dilution effect (figure 61). Ezenwa and colleagues also analyzed data on human cases of West Nile encephalitis and bird diversity for all counties in the State of Louisiana. Again, the results were striking: Louisiana counties with more species of nonpasserine birds had significantly fewer cases of West Nile encephalitis than did counties with fewer nonpasserine species. Ezenwa's group did not find significant correlations between number of passerine species and virus prevalence in either mosquitoes or people.

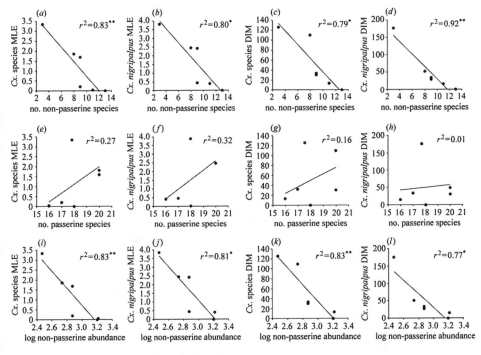

FIGURE 61. Various measures of risk of human exposure to mosquitoes infected with West Nile virus as a function of the species richness of songbirds (passerines) and nonpasserine birds. Both the infection prevalence of mosquitoes (MLE, maximum likelihood estimate) and the density of infected mosquitoes (DIM) strongly, negatively correlated with species diversity of nonpasserines, but were unrelated to species diversity of passerines. *Source:* Ezenwa et al. (2006). Reprinted with permission.

Three follow-up studies have asked whether greater diversity of passerines might reduce West Nile infection risk in other North American sites. Swaddle and Calos (2008) compared bird diversity (both species richness and evenness) in 65 pairs of counties in the United States east of the Mississippi River. Each pair of counties consisted of one county that had reported West Nile encephalitis cases in 2002 ("positive" counties) and an adjacent, matched county that had not ("negative" counties). Using adjacent counties was intended to reduce large-scale geographical differences that might complicate results. These investigators reasoned that, if higher bird diversity reduces disease risk, negative counties should tend to have higher bird diversity than their matched, positive counterparts. To test this hypothesis, Swaddle and Calos made two calculations for each pair of counties: one was the difference in West Nile encephalitis cases per person between counties, and the other was difference in bird diversity between counties. If the dilution effect operates, the researchers expected that the greater the difference between counties in bird diversity, the greater the difference in human incidence. Because West Nile virus can affect bird diversity by killing some species more readily than others (LaDeau et al. 2007), Swaddle and Calos decided to analyze bird diversity data from before (1998) and after (2002) the virus invaded North America. Their analyses demonstrated that West Nile–negative counties had higher bird diversity compared to their positive paired counties. They also showed that the greater the contrast between positive and negative counties in human incidence, the greater the difference in bird diversity. These patterns held regardless of whether bird diversity was measured before or after the invasion of West Nile virus. They estimated that bird diversity explained about 50% of the variation between counties in human incidence of disease.

A strong protective effect of high bird diversity was demonstrated in a continental-scale study by Brian Allan and colleagues (2009). This group analyzed several factors that might influence human incidence of West Nile virus disease in 742 United States counties spread across 38 states over three years. The three main factors of interest were (1) species diversity in the bird community; (2) the total "community competence" in the bird community, which was calculated by multiplying the abundance of each bird species by its reservoir competence, and then adding these together for a total; and (3) human population density. They took a number of statistical precautions to avoid *self-correlations*, another type of *spurious* correlation between variables (that is, the appearance that one variable is causally related to a second variable when in fact it is not). For example, Allan and colleagues were interested in testing whether incidence of West Nile virus disease, represented by the number of cases per 100,000 people, positively correlated with human population density, represented by the number of people per area. Notice, however, that the number of people occurs twice here: as cases per 100,000 people in West Nile virus incidence, and as population per area in population density. To exclude spurious forces, Allan and colleagues used a statistical procedure to remove the potential for *population self-correlation* caused by using human population twice in the same formula (see Allan et al. 2009 for details).

Allan and colleagues (2009) were also concerned that each of the 742 counties might not be independent of one another, which would violate critical assumptions of statistical tests. For example, two adjacent counties might both have high bird diversity and low West Nile disease incidence, but their similarity might occur simply because they are close together and therefore experience similar forces. Allan and colleagues used spatial statistical techniques to estimate the magnitude of this *spatial self-correlation* effect. Lastly, they were concerned that all three of their causal (independent) variables might be interconnected. For example, bird diversity might be lower where human density is higher. And, given that the most competent reservoirs (crows, house finches, house sparrows, robins) seem to dominate in low-diversity communities, community competence would likely be higher where bird diversity is lower. Indeed, they observed a strong negative correlation between community competence and species diversity (but note that this correlation strongly supports a key tenet of the dilution effect). Nevertheless, they statistically accounted for these *intercorrelations* in their analyses.

After such careful treatment of their data, Allan and colleagues (2009) determined that high bird diversity was indeed the strongest and most consistent factor in reducing human incidence of West Nile encephalitis in the United States. People in counties with the highest levels of bird diversity were between 10 and 100 times less likely to become ill with this virus than were people in counties with the lowest levels of bird diversity (figure 62). The result was independent of any effects of human population density on West Nile virus disease.

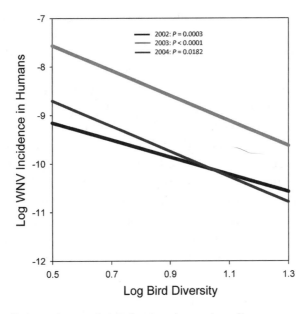

FIGURE 62. Negative correlations between the number of human cases of disease caused by West Nile virus in an American county and the average species diversity of birds in that county as determined by the breeding bird survey. See Allan et al. (2009) for details. *Source:* Ostfeld (2009). Reprinted with permission.

One recent study failed to find support for the dilution effect in West Nile virus dynamics. In 2005 and 2006 Loss and colleagues (2009) sampled mosquito and bird communities in 13 sites within the Chicago metropolitan area in Illinois to assess the relationship between bird diversity and the proportion of *Culex* mosquitoes infected with the virus. This area was chosen because the human population there had experienced a high incidence of West Nile virus encephalitis in 2002, when the virus wave came traveling through the U.S. Midwest. Neither the number of bird species in a site (species richness) nor the proportion of birds testing positive for West Nile virus (seroprevalence) was a significant predictor of mosquito infection prevalence. Loss and colleagues argued that their data supported three of the four necessary conditions for the dilution effect to operate in a vector-borne disease, as laid out by Ostfeld and Keesing (2000a; see chapter 8). They found strong evidence for (1) host-to-vector (horizontal) transmission of the virus, (2) generalized (nonspecific) feeding habits by the mosquito vector, and (3) strong variation among hosts in reservoir competence. The one condition they argued was not met was that the most competent reservoirs tend to dominate in the most species-poor communities. This assertion, however, seems to be contradicted by their finding that mourning doves, northern cardinals, and house finches—three species that preferentially occupy urbanized and suburbanized environments—had the highest seroprevalence values and are known to be among the most competent reservoirs for West Nile virus (Komar et al. 2003, 2005). Instead, it appears that, by limiting their analyses to the highly urbanized environment of metropolitan Chicago, these investigators failed to include a sufficiently high range of bird diversity in their study. Rigorous analysis of the relationship between a *response* variable (here, West Nile virus in mosquitoes) and a putative *causal* variable (bird diversity) requires that both variables show a sufficient *range* of values. Cause-and-effect relationships can be masked when the range is quite modest, as seems to be the case for bird diversity in the Chicago study. In addition, if the wave of West Nile virus in 2002 substantially altered the bird community, which is highly likely based on the studies of LaDeau and colleagues (2007), any prior effect of bird diversity may have been altered or destroyed by the disease itself.

Schistosomiasis

Schistosomiasis is second only to malaria in the magnitude of health and economic costs of a parasitic disease. The disease is endemic to 74 countries and affects about 200 million people, about half of whom live in sub-Saharan Africa (World Health Organization Expert Committee 2002). Schistosomiasis, which has several different versions, is caused by trematode (fluke) parasites that cycle between snail and vertebrate hosts in tropical and subtropical environments. For the species of schistosome that cause human disease, humans act as the *definitive hosts* (those in which sexual reproduction takes place); other mammals act as definitive hosts for other schistosome species. Eggs of schistosomes are released in urine or feces of infected people and hatch into free-swimming forms called *miracidia*. Miracidia seek a freshwater snail as an *intermediate host*, burrow into the snail's foot, and start to replicate, ultimately producing thousands of new parasite forms called *cercariae*. The schistosomes prefer to reside in the gonads of the snail host and can severely damage these tissues, resulting in "parasitic castration" of the snail. Cercariae dribble out of the snail on a daily basis and actively swim about searching for an appropriate definitive host. Once they encounter a human, they attach to the skin and secrete enzymes that make holes, allowing them to enter the blood stream, and then migrate to various tissues, such as the liver, intestines, or bladder, and transform into a sexual stage that produces thousands of eggs.

Each schistosome species that causes disease in humans tends to multiply readily in only one species of intermediate (snail) host, which can be considered analogous to pathogen reservoirs in vector-borne diseases. Other snail species can be invaded by the miracidia but typically do not allow reproduction or the production of cercariae—that is, they are incompetent reservoirs. In the case of the most widespread disease-causing schistosome, *Schistosoma mansoni*, the primary intermediate host consists of snails in the genus *Biomphalaria*. These snails can coexist with several other freshwater snail species, although little is known about factors affecting snail species diversity in freshwater systems with high risk of schistosomiasis.

Recently, Pieter Johnson and colleagues (2009) completed an elegant study to test whether snail diversity might affect human risk of exposure to schistosomiasis, as measured by production of cercariae (the human infectious stage). They built 200 experimental containers in which they placed highly competent schistosome reservoirs (*Biomphalaria glabrata*) either alone or together with incompetent reservoir snails (*Helisoma trivolvis*, *Lymnaea stagnalis*, or both). Abundance of *Biomphalaria* was held constant in each container so that population density of reservoir snails was controlled. Known quantities of *Schistosoma mansoni* miracidia were added to containers and allowed to infect the snails. The key response variables were the proportion of snails that got infected and either the total number of cercariae released by the snails in each container, or the number released per snail. Both of these variables are highly relevant to human risk.

The presence of one or two additional snail species in containers—that is, higher host diversity—dramatically reduced all measures of human risk of exposure to schistosmiasis. When *Biomphalaria* snails were raised alone, 80% became infected with schistosomes, but the presence of either of the other snail species reduced this value to less than 50%. Perhaps even more striking was the observation that *Biomphalaria* snails raised without other snail species released, on average, between two and five times more cercariae per snail than did their counterparts raised with one or two other snail species (figure 63). In an interesting twist, Johnson and colleagues (2009) found that the two additional snails reduced rates of egg production by *Biomphalaria* snails, apparently by competing with them for food. Therefore, higher snail diversity could reduce disease risk by an additional pathway, namely, host regulation by reducing abundance of reservoir hosts (Keesing et al. 2006; see chapter 8). However, when schistosomes were added to the mix, the net effect of adding one or both of the two other snails was to *enhance* snail egg production by *Biomphalaria*. By diverting miracidia away from *Biomphalaria*, these other snails reduced the rate of parasitic castration of *Biomphalaria* and actually increased reproduction in their competitors (Johnson et al. 2009). This research highlights the likely possibility that increases in biodiversity in some disease systems can have multiple and even contrasting effects on disease transmission. Such possibilities would undoubtedly be seen by public health officials as annoying complexities, yet ecologists understand that they are absolutely fundamental to predicting disease risk and intervening effectively.

Rust Diseases of Plants

Diseases of plants cost many billions of dollars every year in lost agricultural, forestry, and ornamental plant production. Two of the most widespread and damaging pathogens of herbaceous plants, especially grasses, are crown rust (*Puccinia coronata*) and stem rust (*P. graminis*) fungi. Although these rusts can attack dozens of grass species to varying degrees, they are among the most frequent and damaging pathogens of perennial ryegrass (*Lolium perenne*), perhaps the most common grass species in temperate-zone turfs and pastures worldwide. Spores of both fungi disperse among plants through rain splash and through air currents. In a carefully designed experimental study in Germany, Roscher and colleagues (2007) addressed

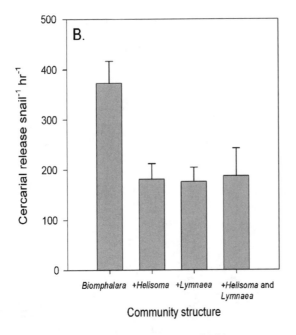

FIGURE 63. The rate of release of infective stages of *Schistosoma mansoni* parasites by their main intermediate hosts, *Biomphalaria* snails. *Biomphalaria* snails were raised either alone or together with one or two other snail species. Increased diversity of snails strongly reduced the release of infective cercariae. *Source:* Johnson et al. (2009). Reprinted with permission.

the role of plant (host) diversity in the intensity of disease caused by crown rust and stem rust. Roscher and colleagues planted several strains (*cultivars*) of perennial ryegrass in a series of 82 field plots 20 meters by 20 meters in size. In 16 of those plots, perennial ryegrass was the only species; in four other groups of either 16 or 14 plots they planted one, three, seven, or fifteen other species in addition to perennial ryegrass, and then in four plots they planted 59 other species plus ryegrass. Seed density was held constant across all of these treatments. The investigators then examined all of the plots for natural infection with the two rust species as the growing season elapsed.

Roscher and colleagues (2007) found a dramatic decline in both the severity of infestation and the proportion of ryegrass plants infested as plant species diversity increased. In fact, for stem rust, some treatments with 16 plant species and all treatments with 60 species drove the pathogen locally extinct (figure 64). All cultivars of perennial ryegrass were strongly protected against both pathogens by increases in plant diversity, although the magnitude of the protective effect varied among cultivars. Roscher and colleagues suggest two different mechanisms by which high diversity

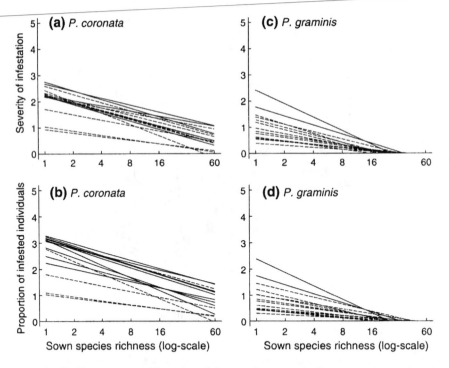

FIGURE 64. Two measures of rust fungal disease of ryegrass *(Lolium perenne)*, severity of infestation and proportion of host plants infested, as a function of the total number of herbaceous plants in experimental field plots containing ryegrass. As plant diversity increased, infestation with disease-causing blast fungi decreased, to the point of extinction in some cases. *Source:* Roscher et al. (2007). Reprinted with permission.

reduced pathogen transmission. They noted that the height and mass of individual ryegrass plants decreased as more plant species co-occurred in the plots. Smaller stature might make individual plants less likely to intercept rain- or air-borne fungal spores. This mechanism is a variation of *host regulation* (Keesing et al. 2006; see chapter 8). In addition, the nearest neighbors of infested ryegrass plants in more diverse plots are more likely to be less susceptible (non-ryegrass) hosts in more diverse than in less diverse plots. These poor reservoirs can intercept dispersing spores but do not provide them an opportunity to multiply. This mechanism is a version of *encounter reduction* (Keesing et al. 2006; see chapter 8). In the past few years, other examples of reduced pathogen transmission with increasing biodiversity (that is, the dilution effect) have been discovered in many disease systems that vary in type of pathogen (viral, bacterial, fungal, metazoan), host (mammal, bird, amphibian, invertebrate, plant), ecosystem (terrestrial, aquatic), and transmission mode (vector-borne and direct).

Commonalities

What do white-footed mice, chipmunks, short-tailed shrews, deer mice, pigmy rice rats, blue jays, robins, grackles, house finches, crows, *Biomphalaria* snails, and perennial ryegrass have in common? For one thing, all of these species tend to be widespread, resilient, even "weedy" species that respond favorably to human-caused disturbances such as habitat destruction and fragmentation. Under disturbed conditions, they are among the most common members of their ecological communities, whereas they tend to be less abundant or even absent when their ecosystems are more pristine. Exactly why these species proliferate in disturbed habitats is not entirely clear. In general, though, species that live fast and die young, that reproduce rapidly and disperse readily, are the ones that invade and do well in disturbed habitats. The ability to proliferate and disperse seems to entail a cost, though. If the organism allocates energy and resources to being highly prolific and mobile, it apparently can't simultaneously invest in longevity, persistence, and resistance to its competitors and predators. In other words, powerful trade-offs constrain the evolution of life-history traits such as reproductive rates, life span, and mobility. So, when habitats are disturbed or frequently altered, as humans tend to do, these "live fast and die young" species are favored, but when disturbances are infrequent or small, they are not. As a consequence, low-diversity communities tend to be dominated by these prolific, mobile species, and in high-diversity communities they are considerably less abundant.

The other obvious feature that all of these species have in common is they are among the most competent reservoirs for important pathogens. Is it simply coincidence that these resilient species with a fast pace of life also tend to be the most competent reservoirs for pathogens? There is essentially no research yet on this topic, but I strongly suspect that the answer is no. Anna Jolles, Felicia Keesing, Andrea Previtali, Rhea Hanselmann, Lynn Martin, and I have been working to develop a theory to explain why resilient species tend to be competent reservoirs for many pathogens. Our current thinking is that, just as these fast-paced, resilient species tend to trade off their ability to stand their ground and fight competitors and predators, so too have they sacrificed their ability to resist pathogens, in order to accelerate reproduction and dispersal.

For any host species, resisting the proliferation of pathogenic microbes can be an energetically expensive proposition. In the case of vertebrates, such resistance is mediated by an adaptive immune system that recognizes specific antigens and launches specific countermeasures, including anti-body production, and this response is energetically costly (Martin et al. 2008, Martin 2009). For species with a relatively short life expectancy, such as mice, chipmunks, and house finches, it may be more advantageous to permit infections rather than to battle them with an "expensive" defense that reduces reproductive output or the ability to disperse. One way of looking at the question is this: If you're a mouse who is likely to die soon in the teeth or beak of a predator, the best way to maximize your fitness might be to quickly produce and scatter your offspring. Focusing your resources on reproducing and dispersing would come at the cost of expensive immune defense, but so what? Why worry about getting a few infections if they're unlikely to kill you before a predator does? Thus, the evolutionary pressures that favor a resilient, fast-paced life history might indirectly result in relaxed immune defenses that allow pathogens to proliferate and persist best in these types of hosts (figure 65).

An alternative explanation for the tendency of resilient, fast-paced host species to be the best pathogen reservoirs is that the pathogen has evolved to be able to proliferate optimally in these types of hosts. In other words,

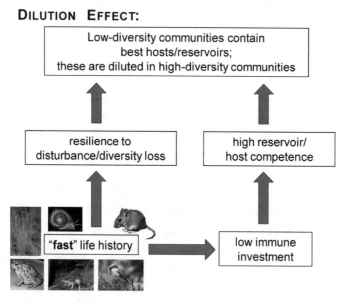

FIGURE 65. Diagram of a possible pathway causing low-diversity communities under habitat fragmentation and degradation to tend to contain species that best amplify disease transmission. Although speculative, such a pathway would explain how high biodiversity provides strong protection against disease risk in different disease systems.

evolution by the pathogen rather than by the host is responsible. In this case, imagine that you're a *Borrelia burgdorferi* bacterium, or a West Nile virus particle. Your only means of producing generations of descendants is to proliferate in a host but not kill it too quickly so that you (or your direct descendants) can be picked up and carried off by a vector. You and your brethren are distributed among dozens to hundreds of different species of hosts because you rely on a vector that is notorious for having varied tastes in hosts—*host generalists*. Blacklegged ticks (for *B. burgdorferi*) and *Culex* mosquitoes (for West Nile virus) will bite pretty much anything with four legs (or two legs and two wings), so by using ticks or mosquitoes for vectors, you and your brethren encounter a very large number of "habitats," that is, host species. As a result, it may be in your best interest to evolve traits that allow you to adjust your replication rates so that they best suit one of those "habitats." (Again, this assumes that trade-offs prevent you from adapting optimally to all of the hosts at the same time.)

If you can only adapt optimally to one or a few hosts, it may be advantageous to adapt to the ones you are most likely to encounter over evolutionary time (which can be fairly short for bacteria and especially viruses). These might be the most resilient, fastest reproducing, most reliably abundant hosts. Adapting to these hosts would involve replicating sufficiently to achieve high blood concentrations, to assure emigration via vector blood meals, but not so much that the host gets very sick or dies quickly. In the case of tick-borne pathogens, it is critical not to badly sicken the host, because host mobility is essential for host–tick contact (that is, hosts move to ticks, and not vice versa). In the case of mosquito-borne pathogens, sickening the host to the degree that it is somewhat lethargic might in fact be optimal. This is because highly mobile mosquitoes don't require highly mobile hosts to ensure contact, and some illness on the part of the host might limit its ability to evade mosquitoes. We might therefore expect tick-borne pathogens to evolve lower virulence in their "preferred" hosts than do mosquito-borne pathogens in their "preferred" hosts (for a more general discussion of this issue, see Ewald 1994).

I do not consider the two hypotheses just described, focusing on host evolution or pathogen evolution, to be mutually exclusive, and indeed, both might operate in the same disease system. It could well be the case that hosts having fast, resilient lifestyles are the most tolerant of infection (the *host immunity* hypothesis) *and* that these are the hosts to which widespread pathogens are most likely to adapt (the *pathogen virulence* hypothesis). It could also be that the host immunity and pathogen virulence hypotheses apply differently to different disease systems. For instance, because each hantavirus tends to specialize on a single species of rodent host, hantavirus populations might not experience a number of different "host habitats" to which they differentially adapt. If so, the pathogen virulence hypothesis would not apply. However, several studies show that nonreservoir species that co-occur with the hantavirus reservoir can be exposed and even infected, even if they don't mount a high viremia (Mills et al. 1997, Klingstrom et al. 2002). This spillover phenomenon is quite commonly observed even for pathogens that are largely specialized on a single host species (Power and Mitchell 2004, Daniels et al. 2007). Therefore, hantaviruses might in fact experience numerous other species besides the specialist host but be able to adapt to only one.

Is Protection from Disease an Ecosystem Function of Biodiversity?

I opened this chapter by describing ecologists' abiding interest in the relationship between biodiversity and the functioning of ecosystems. As is so often the case in newly emerging scientific issues, a debate developed between proponents of two extremes: that biodiversity was fundamentally important to ecosystem functions such that any loss of diversity compromised functioning; and that biodiversity was only weakly involved in ecosystem functioning and was overshadowed by other factors (see Naeem et al. 2009). This polarization has largely subsided as ecologists have agreed on several pivotal issues needing resolution. Below, I describe what these issues are and why they're important. For each issue, I discuss how infectious diseases, especially Lyme disease, fit into this dynamic research focus.

The first of the pivotal issues is *the shape of the relationship between biodiversity and ecosystem functioning.* Dozens of studies have now demonstrated that, as species are added to ecological systems, such ecosystem functions as rates of nutrient cycling, primary production (accumulation of carbon, mainly by plants), and resistance to drought, increase (Naeem et al. 2009). But imagine two extremes describing this increasing functioning with increasing diversity. In one case, every species that gets added to an increasingly diverse community makes a roughly equal contribution to the ecosystem function. This would lead to a *linear* relationship between biodiversity and ecosystem functioning. A critical implication of such a relationship is that every time a species is lost from the system, no matter which species and no matter how high or low the starting diversity, the ecosystem functions more poorly. Such a system would be highly sensitive to biodiversity loss. But a second extreme is that only a few species are necessary for a high-functioning ecosystem, with additional species contributing little if anything. Such a system would be characterized by a *curvilinear* increase to a more or less flat line (*asymptote*) in the zone of moderate to high diversity. The implication here is that the system can function quite well even if it loses a large proportion of its starting biodiversity, and would only collapse if almost all species are lost.

For hantavirus pulmonary syndrome in Oregon, the second extreme seems to represent the relationship between biodiversity and disease risk (Dizney and Ruedas 2009). At very low mammal diversity, disease risk spikes, but above that low level of diversity, disease risk remains largely unchanged. For West Nile virus, rust fungal infections in ryegrass, and Lyme disease, the evidence suggests a pattern intermediate between the two extremes (Schmidt and Ostfeld 2001, Ostfeld and LoGiudice 2003, Ezenwa et al. 2006, Roscher et al. 2007, Allan et al. 2009). The relationship between increasing biodiversity and decreasing disease risk or incidence is clearly curvilinear,[1] although disease risk or incidence continues to decline throughout the range of host biodiversity. In other words, biodiversity loss consistently increases disease risk, but the effects are stronger when going from moderate to low diversity than going from high to moderate diversity. For the other diseases that were reviewed earlier in this chapter, data are insufficient to address the shape of the curve.

The second pivotal issue is *the most appropriate metric of species diversity*. The most commonly used *metric*, or measure, for species diversity is *species richness*, which is simply the number of different species present. Changes in biodiversity are reflected only when species go (at least locally) extinct. Although for some research questions this metric seems appropriate, for others it is inadequate. For understanding the mechanisms by which biodiversity affects disease risk, it seems that species richness is useful but insufficient. One might also need to know how many members of each species there are. For instance, imagine a community consisting of three species—white-footed mice, eastern chipmunks, and short-tailed shrews—with five of each (for a total of 15 animals). Now imagine another community with exactly the same species richness = 3, but with 13 mice, one chipmunk, and one shrew. The effects on Lyme disease risk would be quite different (it would be much higher in this second community) even though species richness didn't change. In ecologists' parlance, the *species evenness* of the first community was high, with equal representation by

---

1. Note that in some of these studies the published curves are straight lines but the axes are scaled logarithmically. If the true arithmetic values of the data were presented on both axes, the curves would be curvilinear.

each, whereas that in the second community was low. Further imagine a third community also having three species and 15 individuals, but now there are five each of mice, opossums, and raccoons. As illustrated in chapter 8, despite identical species richness and maximal species evenness, this community would present vastly lower Lyme disease risk than either of the others. In this case, the importance of *species identity* within the community is demonstrated. When both species identity and species evenness are measured, ecologists can then describe the *species composition* of the community.

Among these metrics of biodiversity, species richness is clearly the easiest to measure, because one need only count the species present in a community. Species composition is the hardest to measure, because the numbers of individuals of each species also must be counted. Species richness is a suitable metric for understanding the relationship between diversity and disease if individuals from each species have a roughly equal impact on disease dynamics. But this rarely seems to be the case. One exception is the strong reduction in West Nile virus prevalence in both mosquitoes and people as the number of nonpasserine bird species increased in Louisiana (Ezenwa et al 2006). This result suggests that all nonpasserines are equivalently poor reservoirs for the virus, and that each species that is added in more diverse communities adds to the pool of poor reservoirs (rather than displacing others). On the other hand, the failure of Loss and colleagues (2009) to find an effect of high species richness of passerines on West Nile virus prevalence in Chicago could have resulted from differences among the passerine species in their effects on virus transmission. Indeed, differences among songbird species in their reservoir competence and attractiveness to mosquitoes have been well demonstrated (see Loss et al. and references therein).

Species evenness would seem to do a better job than species richness at predicting effects on disease transmission, because this metric (usually given by the *Shannon diversity* or *Simpson diversity* index; Krebs 1989) better represents the relative availability of the various species as transmitters or recipients of pathogens. For instance, a bird community with a high Shannon diversity index would present mosquitoes with a large array of potential blood meal hosts (lots of species are well represented), whereas one with a low Shannon diversity index would present a limited selection (only a few species are well represented). The use of this metric of bird diversity, as opposed to species richness, may be why both Swaddle and Calos (2008) and Allan and colleagues (2009) found strong negative correlations between bird diversity and West Nile virus prevalence.

However, because species identity doesn't enter into the computation of these diversity indices, information about these communities important to disease transmission might be lacking. For example, two different bird communities with high Shannon diversity indices could, in theory, present mosquitoes with two different arrays of poor and good reservoirs, depending on which species are present. As I argue earlier in this chapter and in chapter 8, though, it appears that the species that are lost when a community goes from high to low diversity are predictable. This would mean that high Shannon diversity implies a particular constellation of species and low Shannon diversity another.

We learn the most about species diversity when we measure species composition. Despite the time and labor required, measuring species composition might be necessary to fully understand how diversity affects disease transmission (or any other ecosystem function, for that matter). Species composition is of paramount importance when the various species contribute differently to disease transmission and when the sequence of species loss as biodiversity increases or decreases is not orderly and predictable. I am aware of only one study that explicitly compared the impact of species richness versus species composition on disease risk. In this study of Lyme disease risk, LoGiudice and colleagues (2008) estimated vertebrate species richness in 49 forest fragments throughout New Jersey, New York, and Connecticut. They found that the proportion of nymphal black-legged ticks infected with B. burgdorferi decreased with increased species richness, although the effect was statistically weak.

LoGiudice and colleagues (2008) also estimated the relative abundances of each species in each forest fragment and used this information to create a model to predict nymphal infection prevalence in each fragment. Despite some limitations because some data were missing, the use of species composition data allowed this group to predict Lyme disease risk with high accuracy. Quite similar results were obtained by researchers who experimentally examined the relationship between biodiversity and occurrence of a fungal pathogen of prairie plants (Knops et al. 1999, Mitchell et al. 2002, 2003). Although the severity of fungal disease declined with increasing species richness, this relationship was indirect. Study plots with higher species richness had lower densities of the grass species most susceptible to the fungus, and the most direct determinant of fungal severity was the density of that species.

The third pivotal issue is whether species should be considered individually or *lumped into trait groups or functional groups*. In many ecological communities, some species are strongly similar in the ways that they perform ecosystem functions, such as how fast they deplete resources or convert sunlight into stored carbon. Species that are quite similar are considered "functionally redundant" for a particular function.[2] Whenever functional redundancies exist, it seems more appropriate to measure diversity of groups that share traits, or functional groups, rather than diversity of species. To my knowledge, no studies have yet assessed the relevance of this level of diversity for disease risk or incidence. In the case of Lyme disease, one might expect that a diverse group of carnivores (a functional group) that attack small rodents might have a stronger impact in reducing disease risk than would a diverse group of herbivores, which might not directly affect rodent abundances (Ostfeld and Holt 2004, Holt 2008).

The fourth pivotal issue is whether ecosystem functions might be performed better by *monocultures of high-performing species versus diverse polycultures*. Monocultures, which contain just one species—the pinnacle of low diversity—could be better at performing an ecosystem function than are diverse ecosystems, if the species in the monoculture is the most efficient performer of that particular function. For instance, if the ecosystem function of interest is enriching the soil with nitrogen, one might expect a monoculture of nitrogen-fixing legumes (for example, alfalfa) to outperform a diverse mix of pasture plants. Returning to the Lyme disease example, consider two hypothetical ways of reducing disease risk in a habitat containing lots of highly reservoir-competent small mammals. One would be to add a diverse group of other vertebrate hosts that would reduce pathogen transmission and tick survival, and the other would be to add a bunch of opossums (which are particularly poor at transmitting *B. burgdorferi* and good at killing ticks; see chapter 8). It may well be that the opossums would be more effective at reducing disease risk. However, both practical and ethical concerns might undermine enthusiasm for this management technique. Imagine the practical challenges of air-dropping thousands of opossums into an area with endemic Lyme disease. Although feasibility also is a major constraint in managing landscapes to increase vertebrate biodiversity, at least we know some general strategies, such as preserving large, unfragmented tracts, for accomplishing this goal (see chapter 8). Beyond feasibility issues, it might be more ethically justifiable to manage habitats for high diversity than to saturate them with single species, opossums or otherwise.

---

2. Note that rarely, if ever, are species functionally redundant in *all* traits or functions that they perform.

Even if we were to find that in some cases monocultures of very high-performing species are more effective at reducing disease transmission than are diverse polycultures, such a comparison might have little relevance to disease prevention and management. To address prevention, we need to understand how *changes* in biodiversity affect *changes* in disease transmission. In other words, the critical question would seem to be how the burden of disease will change as biodiversity is lost or gained.

The last pivotal issue is *whether biodiversity at levels other than species* is important to ecosystem functioning, including disease transmission. When most ecologists think about biodiversity, counting species is what jumps to mind. But it's important to realize that diversity of entities other than species also can be crucial for ecosystem functioning, including the protection against infectious diseases. For example, instead of counting species, ecologists could count populations within species, or genetically distinct groups (genotypes) belonging to the same species. A few recent studies have shown that the diversity of different genotypes can strongly influence pathogen transmission in the broader ecosystem, and that *genotypic diversity* can act analogously to species diversity.[3]

Imagine a species that is made up of several distinct genotypes (the same way roses are made up of different cultivars with different colors and sizes). If these genotypes differ in their susceptibility to a particular pathogen, in their reservoir competence for that pathogen, or in their suitability for a vector of the pathogen, then the diversity of genotypes might act the same as diversity of species, as described above. Recently, Dennehy and colleagues (2007) described a system in which a bacteriophage (a virus that attacks and kills bacteria) called Φ6 ("fie-six") interacts with its bacterial host, *Pseudomonas phaseolicola*. The "regular" (*wild-type*) genotype of *P. phaseolicola* has small protuberances called *pili* that it uses to attach to plants on which it feeds. But these pili are also the sites that attract Φ6 phages; when the bacterial host draws in its pili, any attached phages enter the cell, replicate, and eventually kill the bacterium. Two naturally occurring mutants of *P. phaseolicola* also exist. One, called *super-piliated*, has lots of pili but never retracts them, so that it attracts many phages but the phages can't penetrate to the interior of the bacterial cell. The other mutant, called *neutral*, has no pili at all and so Φ6 phages are unable to attach.

To ask about the effect of genotypic diversity on phage growth rates, Dennehy and colleagues (2007) subjected monocultures of the wild-type

---

3. One area of biodiversity that is critically important to disease dynamics, but that is beyond the scope of this discussion, is diversity of different types of pathogens within hosts.

Pseudomonas to its Φ6 pathogen—a low-diversity situation—and then added each of the naturally occurring *Pseudomonas* mutant genotypes, creating higher diversity situations. Compared to the wild-type monoculture, a mixed culture of 50% wild type and 50% neutral reduced the abundance of Φ6 phage almost 10-fold. When they presented the phage with a mixture of 50% wild-type and 50% super-piliated *P. phaseolicola*, the phages declined in abundance about 700-fold. Similar to dilution hosts in the Lyme disease or West Nile virus systems, these super-piliated bacteria act as dead-end hosts, attracting pathogens but preventing them from proliferating and attacking the reservoir hosts.

Another example of genotypic diversity reducing disease comes from China's Yunnan Province. The province has a cool, moist climate that is conducive to rice cultivation but also to rice blast fungi (*Magnaporthe grisea*) that attack the plants and undermine yields. A genotype of rice that is particularly vulnerable to rice blast is glutinous rice, grown for various confections. Traditionally, rice farmers throughout Yunnan Province plant vast monocultures of single rice genotypes, and they often experience devastating rice blast epidemics that require repeated applications of fungicides. Youyong Zhu and colleagues (2000) somehow convinced thousands of rice farmers in Yunnan province to plant mixtures of different rice genotypes to test whether an environmentally friendly alternative to fungicides might reduce fungal epidemics and increase yields.

The results of this vast field experiment were astonishing. Simply by planting their glutinous rice genotypes interspersed with other rice varieties, farmers reduced fungal rice blast disease by 94% and increased glutinous rice yields by 89% compared with monocultures. Less susceptible rice varieties intercept fungal spores that might otherwise have landed on glutinous rice plants, thereby reducing transmission (encounter reduction). But perhaps more important, the diverse mixtures of rice genotypes supported a diverse assemblage of fungal pathogens, none of which became very abundant. Each of these pathogens appeared to "vaccinate" rice plants and increase their resistance to multiple pathogens. The end result was that farmers throughout Yunnan Province continued planting polycultures after the experiment ended and ceased having to apply chemical fungicides. This example clearly demonstrates that, when we understand the powerful buffering effect of diversity on disease transmission, we can harness that knowledge to foster environmentally sound management of ecosystems.

10

Embracing Complexity

Biocontrol of Ticks and Lyme Disease

EXOTIC WEEDS IN RANGELANDS AND PASTURES OF THE UNITED STATES dramatically reduce forage quality for grazing livestock and sometimes even poison them. Their economic impact on the livestock industry is estimated at $2 billion U.S. dollars annually, which exceeds the cost of all other pests combined (DiTomaso 2000). One of the major culprits in the western United States and Canada is spotted knapweed, *Centaurea maculosa*. This 1-meter-tall Eurasian transplant is essentially inedible for cattle and sheep, displaces the nutritious grasses favored by these grazers, and makes what remains of these grasses harder to find. Spotted knapweed and its relative diffuse knapweed (*C. diffusa*) also degrade habitat quality for wildlife. Other than their attractive purple or white flowers, these plants have essentially no redeeming features.

Range managers have aggressively sought ways of controlling these exotic weeds. In the 1970s, two species of *Urophora* gall flies were introduced from Eurasia into the western United States as biological control (*biocontrol*) agents. The female gall flies lay eggs inside knapweed flowerheads early in their development, causing the plant to produce tumor-like growths called galls. Apparently the galls are the plant's way of protecting itself against these insect invaders. The investment in gall tissue, however, comes at the expense of investment in reproductive tissue, markedly reducing seed production. Such an effect could stop knapweed from spreading and give native plants a fighting chance to outcompete the invading species.

By the 1970s, the history of spectacular failures in the use of biocontrol was widely known. The biocontrol agents released to tackle exotic pests were themselves exotic (nonnative), and it was difficult to predict how they would behave in their newly colonized areas. The ideal biocontrol agent would attack the targeted pest species and only that species, be very effective at reducing its abundance, and then quietly disappear as it drove its victim extinct. Unfortunately, biocontrol agents don't usually behave this way. One well-known example is the mongooses (*Herpestes javanicus*) that were introduced onto various Caribbean and Pacific islands in an attempt to control rats that were decimating the native birds. The mongooses ate rats but were much more interested in eating the eggs and nestlings of the very birds they were released to protect. In the case of the gall fly introduction for controlling knapweed, biologists spent considerable time asking whether the flies were likely to attack nontarget plants, potentially causing more harm than good. Convinced that the gall flies were well-behaved specialists on knapweed, the biocontrol effort commenced. Indeed, the gall flies behave in their new range exactly as expected—they lay eggs and induce gall formation only in knapweeds, and the galls strongly reduce seed production. Unfortunately, the knapweed species appear quite unhindered by gall flies and have continued to spread dramatically. Moreover, a completely unanticipated, dangerous consequence of the gall fly introduction has emerged—risk of human exposure to deadly hantavirus has increased (Pearson and Callaway 2006). It turns out that the knapweed galls filled with fly larvae are a tasty, nutritious treat for deer mice (*Peromyscus maniculatus*) and provide the mice with an excellent source of food during winter when other foods are scarce. Burgeoning populations of deer mice, which shed hantaviruses in their urine and feces, can cause a major health risk to people. The message here is that biocontrol can be a treacherous path to reducing the impacts of pests and must be considered very carefully before being deployed.

What about ticks? Could biocontrol be used to reduce tick populations and therefore cases of tick-borne disease? To address this question, it would be useful to compile a list of the species that attack ticks in nature. Each species on the list can then be explored for its potential to control ticks and its probability of causing unintended problems, such as attacking nontarget organisms or increasing another ecological problem. Given the enormous burden of disease transmitted by various ticks all over the world, one might expect that such an exploration would have been aggressively pursued. But one would be wrong. Instead, only a partial list of potential biocontrol agents has been amassed, and attempts to assess their suitability for controlling tick numbers have been poorly supported and anemic.

A promising early candidate as a control agent for blacklegged ticks was the helmeted guinea fowl, *Numida meleagris* (figure 66). Flocks of these omnivorous African natives are kept by many American property owners for meat, as pets, as "watchdogs" (they vocalize loudly when disturbed), and, more recently, as tick control agents. Based on a single, modest study (Duffy et al. 1992), this bird has achieved cult status as a consumer of ticks and protector of people against Lyme disease. Duffy and his coauthors, including supermodel Christy Brinkley, studied the effects of guinea fowl on ticks on Ms. Brinkley's lawn in the Hamptons on Long Island, New York. They used small fenced areas either to exclude the birds or to concentrate them, and they compared numbers of ticks inside versus outside the fenced areas. They found that adult blacklegged ticks were more abundant where the birds were fenced out and surmised that guinea fowl were eating ticks. Unfortunately, the impact of guinea fowl on ticks was limited to the adult stage and to lawn habitats; adult ticks transmit few cases of Lyme disease (nymphs are the primary culprit), and lawns are a much lower risk habitat than forests or forest–field edges (reviewed by Ostfeld et al. 2006c).

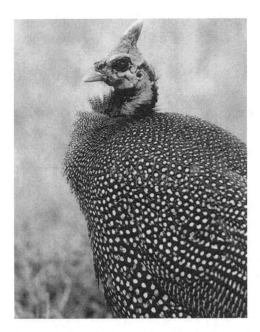

FIGURE 66. A helmeted guinea fowl, *Numida meleagris. Source*: Ostfeld et al. (2006c). Reprinted with permission.

Led by undergraduate student Amber Price, my research group followed the study of Duffy and colleagues by asking whether tick populations were lower on properties that maintained free-ranging guinea fowl than on those that did not. Price identified 10 properties in a highly Lyme-disease-endemic portion of Dutchess County, New York, that maintained free-ranging guinea fowl and matched each of these with a nearby, similar property that had never had guinea fowl (or any other fowl). She then sampled nymphal and adult blacklegged ticks in the middle of lawns, the edges of lawns near the surrounding forest, and just inside the forest. Although adult ticks were significantly less abundant on properties with guinea fowl, this effect was modest (about a 30% reduction) and was limited to the forest edge. Abundances of nymphal ticks were not significantly different between properties with and without guinea fowl, suggesting that the birds are unable to protect humans from exposure to tick-borne disease. Publication of these sobering results several years ago (Ostfeld et al. 2006c) has not appeared to dampen enthusiasm for this method of controlling ticks.

My research group also tested whether a native fowl, the wild turkey (*Meleagris gallopavo*), might consume ticks and reduce their populations. Wild turkeys are increasing in numbers and geographic range (Kennamer et al. 1992) and are known to be generalist consumers that include various arthropods in their diets. Dave Lewis and I established replicate field enclosures in forests at the Cary Institute of Ecosystem Studies in Millbrook, New York, using plastic snow fencing and purchased five captive-bred wild turkeys from a local grower (Ostfeld and Lewis 1999). We placed known numbers of adult blacklegged ticks inside each of six enclosures and allowed them to acclimate for several days. We then introduced the turkeys into three of the enclosures and allowed them to forage for several hours (the birds began scratching and pecking within seconds after being released). They were then returned to their turkey coop, and this process was repeated for several days. Comparison of the enclosures with and without turkeys revealed that the birds did not consume adult ticks, although they readily ate the acorns that we had also deployed. In a related project examining whether wild turkeys were competent reservoirs for *Borrelia burgdorferi*, Lewis and I placed first nymphal and then larval ticks on the birds to see if turkeys got infected from the nymphs and then transmitted infections to the larvae. To collect the ticks after they finished feeding on the birds, we placed pans of water (ironically, these were modified turkey basting pans) beneath the cages that held the turkeys. To our surprise, we collected only a tiny fraction of the ticks that we had placed on the animals; the turkeys had apparently consumed all the others while grooming (Ostfeld and Lewis 1999). At the time, we considered this part of the experiment a failure and realized only years later that the ability of hosts to kill ticks by grooming and swallowing them might be critical in regulating tick populations (Keesing et al. 2009).

It would seem that a variety of native vertebrates, including turkeys, opossums, and gray squirrels (see chapter 8), can act as powerful natural enemies of ticks by killing those that attempt to feed on the host's blood. But only weak evidence supports these vertebrates' abilities to kill ticks that are on the forest floor or on understory vegetation, where they spend more than 95% of their lives. What happens to ticks while they are on the forest floor digesting a blood meal, remaining quiescent for months at a time, or seeking a host, is a huge mystery. We know that only a small fraction of the ticks in each life stage survives to the next stage, but we have very little information on what kills them. I argue in chapter 5 that scant evidence supports the notion that climatic conditions are responsible for these poor survival rates from one stage to the next, although much testing of climate effects remains to be done. What if ticks were regularly stalked by microscopic forest floor creatures that can attack and kill them?

Such creatures are known to exist. *Bacillus thuringiensis* bacteria, which are famous for their ability to kill insect pests, including mosquitoes, also kill ticks (Zhioua et al. 1999). Unfortunately, these bacteria need to be ingested by the tick in order to cause damage or death. Because ticks eat only one thing—blood—our ability to deliver the bacteria to where they need to go is severely limited, and the prospects for using *B. thuringiensis* as a biocontrol agent seem dim. Similarly, microscopic nematode worms in the families Steinernematidae and Heterorhabditidae, including commercial formulations for controlling insect pests, are able to kill ticks. These nematodes either secrete digestive enzymes that assist them in drilling through the tick's cuticle, or they invade through natural orifices such as the anogenital pore. Once inside a tick, the worms release the bacteria that they carry around, and these bacteria return the favor by digesting the tick's tissues, releasing nutrients for the nematodes to consume (Zhioua et al. 1995). However, the ability of these nematodes to control tick populations in nature appears quite limited. Apparently only engorged adult ticks are susceptible to attack by the nematodes, leaving critically important life stages invulnerable. Also, the nematodes apparently are unable to reproduce within ticks and require other hosts to fulfill their life cycles (Samish and Glazer 2001).

The forest floor microbes that show the most promise in controlling tick populations are fungi. Two fungal species—*Metarhizium anisopliae* and *Beauveria bassiana*—have been tested experimentally on ticks and do a good job killing various species of tick, including blacklegged ticks (reviewed by Ostfeld et al. 2006c) (figure 67). In addition to killing ticks outright, these fungi can cause ticks to feed on host blood more poorly, resulting in lighter body mass after feeding, and reduce their success in molting into the next stage or laying eggs (Hornbostel et al. 2004). To test the ability of these fungi to kill or sicken ticks, researchers take advantage of commercial "biocide" products that are labeled for use against pest insects such as termites, carpenter ants, and agricultural pests. The commercial products are not intended for use against ticks, but like many chemical insecticides, they do a reasonable job of killing many arthropods in addition to the target species (Ginsberg et al. 2002). Both *M. anisopliae*

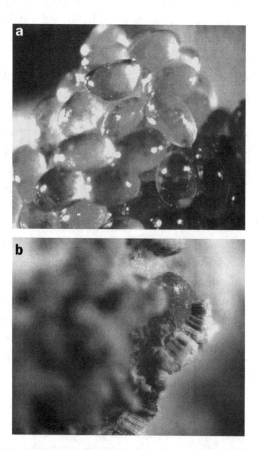

FIGURE 67. The fungus *Metarhizium anisopliae* attacking eggs of a blacklegged tick (bottom). Fungus-free eggs are shown in the top photo. This fungus infects all life stages of many species of tick, sickening or killing them. *Source:* Ostfeld et al. (2006c). Reprinted with permission.

and *B. bassiana* are genetically quite diverse, leading to the possibility that some genetic strains might be more highly lethal to ticks than are the commercial strains (Freimoser et al. 2003, 2005). Fungal biocontrol agents deployed against ticks would be more effective and safer if they consisted of genetic strains that were both highly lethal and specific to ticks. It seems likely that such strains exist in nature waiting to be discovered.

A fascinating recent study by Tuininga and colleagues (2009) surveyed naturally occurring fungi on ticks and in the soil and leaf litter within tick habitats using molecular diagnostic methods. By swabbing ticks and dirt to obtain DNA samples, these researchers found at least 19 species of potentially arthropod-killing (*entomopathogenic*) fungi on the cuticles of ticks or in their forest floor environments. About one-third of the samples these researchers took from ticks, soil, and insect "bait" (larvae of *Gallaria mellonella* beetles) contained potentially entomopathogenic fungi; in contrast, very few leaf litter samples tested positive. Apparently, scores of microscopic natural enemies lurk in the soils where ticks dwell, and clearly ticks get exposed to these pathogens. The potentially pathogenic fungi listed by Tuininga's group provides an excellent point of departure for delving into the community ecology of soil fungi and their arthropod victims.

How lethal is each of the fungal species to ticks? How many arthropod species other than ticks does it attack? Do the most lethal tick-killing species require ticks for propagation, or can they be fostered by providing bait insects that might maintain them when ticks are scarce? How can contact rates between ticks and their pathogens be maximized? Of course, the lessons from failed biocontrol studies should dictate an additional set of questions: Might some entomopathogenic fungi intensify their attacks on nontarget arthropods when ticks become scarce? Will promoting some species or genotypes of fungi suppress others that might help control ticks? Do the various entomopathogenic fungi competitively interfere with each other, or might some species facilitate attack by others? By unraveling the community ecology of ticks and microbes in forest soils we might unearth new, ecologically sound methods of controlling tick populations.

11

Embracing Complexity

In Pursuit of Emerging Infectious Diseases

I LIVE IN THE HUDSON RIVER VALLEY OF NEW YORK STATE, LAND OF Frederick Church vistas, the Catskill Mountains, and rolling, forested hills bisected by rocky streams. George Washington encamped here with his troops during the Revolutionary War. The Culinary Institute of America, Woodstock, Bard and Vassar colleges, and the Dia Museum of Contemporary Art provide cultural riches to the area. Small villages and hamlets dot the landscape, with strip malls and traffic congestion limited to the small cities of Poughkeepsie, Kingston, and Beacon. The biggest employer is International Business Machines (IBM), with health care, higher education, tourism, and agriculture among the other top employers. Median family income in 2003 was $68,000; rates of unemployment and poverty are comparatively low. But the bucolic scenery, diverse culture, and high standard of living are deceptive, because this area is also the setting of wave after wave of emerging infectious diseases. Our culturally and economically privileged lifestyle does not protect us from these diseases and, indeed, might exacerbate them.

Lyme disease emerged here in the mid to late 1980s, and case numbers have grown explosively since then. Human granulocytic anaplasmosis (formerly called granulocytic ehrlichiosis)—another disease vectored by the blacklegged tick—emerged a decade later and has increased dramatically in incidence up through the present. At about the same time, another tick-borne disease, human monocytic ehrlichiosis, began to invade the area. Cases of the tick-borne, malaria-like disease babesiosis have gone from zero to 60 within the past five years. Mosquito-borne diseases are also repeatedly arising in this area, including eastern equine encephalitis, Cache Valley virus, and West Nile encephalitis in wildlife and humans. For these viral diseases, human fatality rates can be as high as 35%. As I write this (late May 2009), 12,950 cases of swine flu (influenza A:H1N1) have been reported from 46 countries scattered throughout the world; two of the victims live in Dutchess County.

Although these diseases differ greatly in lethality and in the numbers of people afflicted, together they present an enormous health threat to human populations locally, regionally, and in some cases internationally. What steps have been taken to reduce the burden of these diseases? Diagnosis and treatment of most of these diseases remain quite problematic. Blood tests can be inaccurate, and symptoms can be too generalized to allow clinical diagnosis. Antimicrobial drugs aimed at *Babesia* and viruses have limited efficacy or are not prescribed. Not a single vaccine is available for human use for any one of these diseases.[1] Guidelines for avoidance and prevention are rudimentary at best.

It is far from the case, though, that scientists have stood idly by watching these diseases sicken and kill many thousands of people. Most, if not all, of these pathogens have been characterized in excruciating molecular detail. The entire genome of *Borrelia burgdorferi* has been sequenced. Different genetic strains of these viral and bacterial pathogens have been described, and trees describing evolutionary relationships have been constructed. Genetic loci responsible for pathogenicity and other loci involved in evading the host's immune system and finding the right target cell types have been identified and characterized. Similarly, the molecular biology of mosquito and tick vectors that permit efficient transmission of the pathogens has been vigorously pursued. Genes that cause the vectors to be permissive to the pathogen have been identified, and mutant vectors without these genes have been created. To be sure, these lines of scientific inquiry are promising. Yet to date, their contributions to prevention, diagnosis, and cure have been limited, to say the least. This is despite the many millions of dollars and uncounted person-hours invested over the years. We still use decades-old, highly imperfect blood tests to detect Lyme disease and still treat it with antibiotics that have been in use since the early 1960s or before.

In this book I have argued that ecological knowledge has been grossly underused to reduce the burden of disease. Why should this be so, especially

---

1. Vaccines targeted for domestic animals exist for some of these diseases, for example, a Lyme disease vaccine for dogs and West Nile virus and eastern equine encephalitis vaccines for horses.

for Lyme disease, which is one of the ecologically best-characterized vector-borne diseases in the world? With the benefit of 20:20 hindsight, the missteps in pursuing ecological understanding of Lyme disease risk are apparent. The early misidentification and mischaracterization of the tick vector led to an oversimplified version of the tick life cycle and inadequate list of important hosts. Naive extrapolations of laboratory results (for example, tick sensitivity to low humidity) led to inadequate models of the physical, abiotic factors that might limit tick distributions. A pervasive reductionist, parts-make-up-the-whole philosophy of scientific pursuit led to an unfortunate narrowing of the list of candidate species, habitats, and processes involved in determining risk. Ironically, more relevant, holistic, whole-is-greater-than-the-parts information exists for Lyme disease than for any of the other emerging diseases listed above. For example, despite the emergence of babesiosis roughly simultaneously with Lyme disease, we still lack even a remotely comprehensive list of reservoir hosts for the causative agent. The same is true of the causative agents of human granulocytic anaplasmosis, human monocytic ehrlichiosis, and eastern equine encephalitis. More work remains to be done for West Nile virus as well. For the mosquito-borne encephalitis viruses, we don't yet know the proportion of transmission events or of human cases caused by the various mosquito species known to be competent vectors. And we don't know whether the availability of hosts in general, or of particular species of hosts, or of predators, or of breeding sites, regulates vector abundances.

We don't have this information because we haven't asked the questions. Instead, we, as a scientific community, have prioritized other questions over these ecological ones. We have also been satisfied with incomplete ecological knowledge (partial lists of reservoirs, vectors, habitats, and so on) even when it's evident that such rudimentary knowledge can lead to ineffective control efforts (see chapter 6). The molecular approaches have been no more successful (and probably less so) in leading to preventive interventions, yet interest in and support for such pursuits continue to accelerate. This is fine. But until we can create, mass-produce, and properly distribute safe, cheap, and effective vaccines for each emerging pathogen, or replace wild vector populations with genetically engineered ones unable to transmit pathogens, ecological knowledge will remain indispensible. In other words, ecological knowledge will always be crucial.

As zoonotic diseases continue to emerge and reemerge all over the world, the need to replace old reductionist paradigms will only increase. The fact that infectious diseases are ecological systems can hardly be overemphasized. Once we recognize this fact, we come to realize that identifying the organisms involved, even in exquisite detail, is not enough; instead, *interactions among organisms* determine disease risk. Once the critical step of identifying the pathogen has been taken, we must cast a broader net to identify where in nature the pathogen comes from, what regulates its abundance and distribution, and what influences its contact rate with important hosts, including us. The guiding principle underlying this pursuit should be that pathogens, reservoirs, and vectors are embedded within ecological communities that influence their abundances, distributions, and contact rates. Realizing that all these species are part of interaction webs does not mean that we should embrace a fluffy mindset represented by the platitude that "everything is connected to everything else." Instead, we understand enough about ecological communities to suspect which species will be most strongly interconnected, and by what mechanisms. Not all species interactions are equal, and many can be reasonably ignored; however, the decision to ignore species and interactions should be guided by data showing that they are inconsequential, not by intuition alone.

A key place to start is to ask to what degree the pathogen, its vector (if one or more are involved), and its hosts are generalized versus specialized. If the pathogen is generalized, meaning it can persist in many different species of host, we need to determine the contributions of those hosts to pathogen proliferation. Focusing on a small subset of such hosts will lead to incomplete and potentially misleading information. If the vector is generalized (that is, feeds on many different host species), effort must be made to ask how much each host contributes to vector abundance and distribution patterns. For the hosts with the numerically dominant effects on pathogen and vector dynamics, it will be important to identify the main factors that regulate their numbers. This will include both "bottom-up" effects of food and other resources and "top-down" impacts of predators and pathogens. The relative strengths of specific biotic and abiotic (for example, climatic) factors need to be determined.

These tasks are certainly challenging, but we can still make rapid progress on a research budget much smaller than those of many grants devoted to sequencing the genome of a particular pathogen or vector. A broad survey of potential hosts, using field reconnaissance or blood-meal analysis (see, for example, Kilpatrick et al. 2006b), can produce a candidate list for further exploration. Combined field and laboratory studies can generate estimates of critical factors such as the rate at which hosts shed pathogens, the number (or proportion) of vectors that feed on each species, the number of vectors killed attempting to feed on each species, and the number that get infected feeding on each species. Further field studies can estimate where in the environment each species occurs and in what numbers.

Newly emerging pathogens are highly likely to spread. Predicting where they will disperse and how fast is critically important to protecting public health. For pathogens that are contagious among humans, such as H1N1 flu viruses or SARS virus, spread is strongly influenced by patterns of human travel. The age of globalization has facilitated almost instantaneous intercontinental jumps by these pathogens, resulting in the establishment of new endemic areas quite distant from the sites of initial emergence. Rampant travel can also produce epidemics and pandemics that would have been highly unlikely in prior eras. The technology that accompanies globalization, however, can also produce mitigation strategies; witness the use of devices in airports that detect passengers with a fever, allowing them to be quarantined.

For zoonotic pathogens that are not contagious, immediate dangers of rampant spread are lessened, but prospects for future spread might be heightened and less amenable to simple controls like quarantines. The habit of lurking within nonhuman hosts and within vectors makes these pathogens less predictable and less controllable. All of the tick-borne and mosquito-borne diseases mentioned in this chapter arose elsewhere, and the Hudson River Valley was one of the many locations unfortunate enough to be in the path of the spreading waves. All of them continue to spread in ways that are largely unpredictable. Public health officials are unable to control the spread simply by quarantining suspected victims or curtailing human travel. As a consequence, residents of newly invaded areas are unaware of the novel health threat, their health care providers are slow to diagnose and treat the illness, and the burden of disease can be devastating.

The lessons learned from Lyme disease can help us improve our ability to predict spread, warn people of impending threats, and provide information on avoiding risk. Such lessons include the following. Detecting the presence versus absence of the vector provides only the most rudimentary information for understanding risk. Instead, we need to estimate the abundance of the vector, or some similar metric of probability of human encounter, and the proportion of vectors infected with the pathogen. We need to be inclusive, rather than exclusive, in our studies of hosts and reservoirs if we want to be able to predict where risk will be high and where it will be low. Certain landscape elements such as rivers, major highways, and urban centers might prevent or slow the dispersal of key hosts or the vectors themselves; therefore, we need to understand animal dispersal patterns in real landscapes. Human-caused disturbances such as habitat fragmentation and destruction can reduce or eliminate certain animal species while facilitating others. Because some of these species increase disease risk whereas others decrease it, we need to know which species are likely to drop out and which will explode. Overly simplistic climate models can produce nonsensical predictions about future spread of diseases. This is more likely to occur when the model incorrectly assumes that a dynamic, rapidly changing situation is in steady state, when only a subset of important climatic variables (or unsubstantiated variables) is included in the model, and when critical contributors to disease risk such as hosts are excluded. To be useful, the climate models must be based, at least in part, on an understanding of the mechanisms by which climate variables affect pathogens, vectors, hosts, or their habitats. Therefore, we should avoid being seduced by the availability of increasingly better, higher resolution, and more accurate remote-sensing data (for example, from satellites) on conditions on the ground. Direct data showing how the organisms are affected by specific climatic variables will remain indispensible for repudiating spurious correlations in remote-sensing data.

In the heady days of the 1960s and 1970s, mainstream public health experts in the developed world became convinced that, with the newly developed arsenal of vaccines and powerful antimicrobial drugs, infectious disease was in full retreat. Militaristic sloganeering the likes of "vanquishing the enemy," "wiping out pathogens," "annihilation," and "victory" was rampant. Currently, no credible public health official that I'm aware of claims that we are winning the war against infectious diseases. Unfortunately, though, the dominant militaristic paradigm has evolved into a firefighter mentality. Once the fire of disease has ignited, we deploy the most powerful hoses we can find, take aim, and open the spigot. It usually works but leaves us little the wiser about where and when the sparks will next ignite. Sitting back in the proverbial fire station (read laboratory) waiting for the next emergency is insufficient. Instead, I hope that we can convert our outmoded militaristic attitudes about the infectious enemy into diplomacy. We need to understand infectious disease so intimately that we can coax it to drop its arms. Ecologists might not want to think of themselves as diplomats, but that's what we need to be.

Literature Cited

Allan, B. F., F. Keesing, and R. S. Ostfeld. 2003. Effect of forest fragmentation on Lyme disease risk. Conservation Biology 17:267–272.

Allan, B. F., R. B. Langerhans, W. A. Ryberg, W. J. Landesman, N. W. Griffin, R. S. Katz, B. J. Oberle, M. R. Schutzenhofer, K. N. Smyth, A. de St. Maurice, L. Clark, K. R. Crooks, D. E. Hernandez, R. G. McLean, R. S. Ostfeld, and J. M. Chase. 2009. Ecological correlates of risk and incidence of West Nile virus in the United States. Oecologia 158:699–708.

Anderson, J. F., and L. A. Magnarelli. 1980. Vertebrate host relationships and distribution of ixodid ticks (Acari: Ixodidae) in Connecticut, USA. Journal of Medical Entomology 17:314–323.

Anderson, J. F., and L. A. Magnarelli. 1984. Avian and mammalian hosts for spirochete-infected ticks and insects in a Lyme disease focus in Connecticut. Yale Journal of Biology and Medicine 57:627–641.

Anderson, J. F., L. A. Magnarelli, W. Burgdorfer, and A. G. Barbour. 1983. Spirochetes in *Ixodes dammini* and mammals from Connecticut. American Journal of Tropical Medicine and Hygiene 32:818–824.

Anderson, R. M., and R. M. May. 1979. Population biology of infectious diseases: part 1. Nature 280:361–367.

Anderson, R. M., and R. M. May. 1981. The population dynamics of micro-parasites and their invertebrate hosts. Philosophical Transactions of the Royal Society of London, Series B, Biological Sciences 291:451–524.

Antonovics, J., Y. Iwasa, and M. P. Hassell. 1995. A generalized model of parasitoid, venereal, and vector-based transmission processes. American Naturalist 145:661–675.

Armstrong, P. M., L. R. Brunet, A. Spielman, and S. R. Telford. 2001. Risk of Lyme disease: perceptions of residents of a Lone Star tick-infested community. Bulletin of the World Health Organization 79:916–925.

Barbour, A. G., and D. Fish. 1993. The biological and social phenomenon of Lyme disease. Science 260:1610–1616.

Benach, J. L., E. M. Bosler, J. P. Hanrahan, J. L. Coleman, G. S. Habicht, T. F. Bast, D. J. Cameron, J. L. Ziegler, A. G. Barbour, W. Burgdorfer, R. Edelman, and R. A. Kaslow. 1983. Spirochetes isolated from the blood of two patients with Lyme disease. New England Journal of Medicine 308:740–742.

Bergstrom, D. M., A. Lucieer, K. Kiefer, J. Wasley, L. Belbin, T. K. Pedersen, and S. L. Chown. 2009. Indirect effects of invasive species removal devastate World Heritage Island. Journal of Applied Ecology 46:73–81.

Bertrand, M. R., and M. L. Wilson. 1996. Microclimate-dependent survival of unfed adult *Ixodes scapularis* (Acari: Ixodidae) in nature: life cycle and study design implications. Journal of Medical Entomology 33:619–627.

Bi, P., S. Tong, K. Donald, K. Parton, and J. Ni. 2002. Climatic, reservoir and occupational variables and the transmission of haemorrhagic fever with renal syndrome in China. International Journal of Epidemiology 31:189–193.

Biodiversity Project. 2002. Americans and Biodiversity: New Perspectives for 2002. Belden Russonello and Stewart Research and Communications, Washington, DC. Available: http://www.biodiversityproject.org/docs/publicopinionresearch/americansandbiodiversitynewperspectivesfor2002.PDF.

Bosler, E. M., J. L. Coleman, J. L. Benach, D. A. Massey, J. P. Hanrahan, W. Burgdorfer, and A. G. Barbour. 1983. Natural distribution of the *Ixodes dammini* spirochete. Science 220:321–322.

Brack, V., Jr. 2006. Short-tailed shrews (*Blarina brevicauda*) exhibit unusual behavior in an urban environment. Urban Habitats 4:127–132.

Brei, B., J. S. Brownstein, J. E. George, J. M. Pound, J. A. Miller, T. J. Daniels, R. C. Falco, K. C. Stafford, T. L. Schulze, T. N. Mather, J. F. Carroll, and D. Fish. 2009. Evaluation of the United States Department of Agriculture northeast area-wide tick control project by meta-analysis. Vector-Borne and Zoonotic Diseases 9:423–430.

Brisson, D., and D. E. Dykhuizen. 2004. ospC diversity in *Borrelia burgdorferi*: different hosts are different niches. Genetics 168:713–722.

Brisson, D., D. E. Dykhuizen, and R. S. Ostfeld. 2008. Conspicuous impacts of inconspicuous hosts on the Lyme disease epidemic. Proceedings of the Royal Society, Series B, Biological Sciences 275:227–235.

Brook, B. W., N. S. Sodhi, and C. J. A. Bradshaw. 2008. Synergies among extinction drivers under global change. Trends in Ecology and Evolution 23:453–460.

Brownstein, J. S., T. R. Holford, and D. Fish. 2003. A climate-based model predicts the spatial distribution of the Lyme disease vector *Ixodes scapularis* in the United States. Environmental Health Perspectives 111:1152–1157.

Brownstein, J. S., D. K. Skelly, T. R. Holford, and D. Fish. 2005. Forest fragmentation predicts local scale heterogeneity of Lyme disease risk. Oecologia 146:469–475.

Brucechwatt, L. J. 1987. Malaria and its control—present situation and future prospects. Annual Review of Public Health 8:75–110.

Brunner, J. L., and R. S. Ostfeld. 2008. Multiple causes of variable tick burdens on small-mammal hosts. Ecology 89:2259–2272.

Burgdorfer, W. 1989. Vector host relationships of the Lyme disease spirochete, *Borrelia burgdorferi*. Rheumatic Disease Clinics of North America 15:775–787.

Burgdorfer, W., A. G. Barbour, S. F. Hayes, J. L. Benach, E. Grunwaldt, and J. P. Davis. 1982. Lyme disease—a tick-borne spirochetosis. Science 216:1317–1319.

Burgdorfer, W., S. F. Hayes, and D. Corwin. 1989. Patho-physiology of the Lyme disease spirochete, *Borrelia burgdorferi*, in ixodid ticks. Reviews of Infectious Diseases 11:S1442–S1450.

Burke, G. S., S. K. Wikel, A. Spielman, S. R. Telford, K. McKay, P. J. Krause, and the Tick-Borne Infection Study Group: R. Pollack, P. Tomas, S. Tahan, D. Christianson, T. V. Rajan, P. Baute, L. Closter, J. Miller, R. Ryan, F. Dias, P. Fall, T. Urso, C. Abreu, and J. Covault. 2005. Hypersensitivity to ticks and Lyme disease risk. Emerging Infectious Diseases 11:36–41.

Burks, C. S., R. L. Stewart, G. R. Needham, and R. E. Lee. 1996. The role of direct chilling injury and inoculative freezing in cold tolerance of *Amblyomma americanum*, *Dermacentor variabilis* and *Ixodes scapularis*. Physiological Entomology 21:44–50.

Calisher, C. H., J. J. Root, J. N. Mills, and B. J. Beaty. 2002. Assessment of ecologic and biologic factors leading to Hantavirus pulmonary syndrome, Colorado, USA. Croatian Medical Journal 43:330–337.

Carey, A. B., W. L. Krinsky, and A. J. Main. 1980. *Ixodes dammini* (Acari, Ixodidae) and associated Ixodid ticks in south-central Connecticut, USA. Journal of Medical Entomology 17:89–99.

Carroll, J. F., P. C. Allen, D. E. Hill, J. M. Pound, J. A. Miller, and J. E. George. 2002. Control of *Ixodes scapularis* and *Amblyomma americanum* through use of the "4-poster" treatment device on deer in Maryland. Experimental and Applied Acarology 28:289–296.

Carroll, J. F., J. M. Pound, J. A. Miller, and A. Kramer. 2008. Reduced interference by gray squirrels with 4-poster deer treatment bait stations by using timed-release bait. Journal of Vector Ecology 33:325–332.

Ceballos, G., and P. R. Ehrlich. 2002. Mammal population losses and the extinction crisis. Science 296:904–907.

Centers for Disease Control and Prevention. 2008. Surveillance for Lyme disease—United States, 1992–2006. MMWR Morbidity and Mortality Weekly Report 57:1–9.

Centers for Disease Control and Prevention. 2009. West Nile virus. Available at: http://www.cdc.gov/ncidod/dvbid/westnile/index.htm

Centers for Disease Control and Prevention. 2010. Emergency preparedness and response: Bioterrorism agents/diseases. Available at: http://www.bt.cdc.gov/agent/agentlist-category.asp

Childs, J. E. 2009. Low-tech versus high-tech approaches for vector-borne disease control. Vector-Borne and Zoonotic Diseases 9:355–356.

Clay, C. A., E. M. Lehmer, S. S. Jeor, and M. D. Dearing. 2009. Sin Nombre virus and rodent species diversity: a test of the dilution and amplification hypotheses. PLoS ONE 4:e6467.

Clement, J., J. Vercauteren, W. W. Verstraeten, G. Ducoffre, J. M. Barrios, A. M. Vandamme, P. Maes, and M. Van Ranst. 2009. Relating increasing hantavirus incidences to the changing climate: the mast connection. International Journal of Health Geographics 8:1.

Connally, N. P., H. S. Ginsberg, and T. N. Mather. 2006. Assessing peridomestic entomological factors as predictors for Lyme disease. Journal of Vector Ecology 31:364–370.

Cromley, E. K., M. L. Cartter, R. D. Mrozinski, and S. H. Ertel. 1998. Residential setting as a risk factor for Lyme disease in a hyperendemic region. American Journal of Epidemiology 147:472–477.

Daniels, P. W., K. Halpin, A. Hyatt, and D. Middleton. 2007. Infection and disease in reservoir and spillover hosts: determinants of pathogen emergence. Pages 113–131 *in* Wildlife and Emerging Zoonotic Diseases: The Biology, Circumstances and Consequences of Cross-Species Transmission (J. E. Childs, J. S. Mackenzie, and J. A. Richt, editors). Current Topics in Microbiology and Immunology no. 315. Springer, Berlin.

Daniels, T. J., and D. Fish. 1995. Effect of deer exclusion on the abundance of immature *Ixodes scapularis* (Acari, Ixodidae) parasitizing small and medium-sized mammals. Journal of Medical Entomology 32:5–11.

Daniels, T. J., D. Fish, and R. C. Falco. 1991. Evaluation of host-targeted acaricide for reducing risk of Lyme disease in southern New York State. Journal of Medical Entomology 28:537–543.

Deblinger, R. D., and D. W. Rimmer. 1991. Efficacy of a permethrin-based acaricide to reduce the abundance of *Ixodes dammini* (Acari: Ixodidae). Journal of Medical Entomology 28:708–711.

Deblinger, R. D., M. L. Wilson, D. W. Rimmer, and A. Spielman. 1993. Reduced abundance of immature *Ixodes dammini* (Acari: Ixodidae) following incremental removal of deer. Journal of Medical Entomology 30:144–150.

Dennehy, J. J., N. A. Friedenberg, Y. W. Yang, and P. E. Turner. 2007. Virus population extinction via ecological traps. Ecology Letters 10:230–240.

Dennis, D. T., T. S. Nekomoto, J. C. Victor, W. S. Paul, and J. Piesman. 1998. Reported distribution of *Ixodes scapularis* and *Ixodes pacificus* (Acari : Ixodidae) in the United States. Journal of Medical Entomology 35:629–638.

Desai, S., U. van Treeck, M. Lierz, W. Espelage, L. Zota, A. Sarbu, M. Czerwinski, M. Sadkowska-Todys, M. Avdicova, J. Reetz, E. Luge, B. Guerra, K. Nockler, and A. Jansen. 2009. Resurgence of field fever in a temperate country: an epidemic of leptospirosis among seasonal strawberry harvesters in Germany in 2007. Clinical Infectious Diseases 48:691–697.

Despommier, D. 2001. West Nile Story. Apple Trees Productions, LLC, New York.

Dister, S. W., D. Fish, S. M. Bros, D. H. Frank, and B. L. Wood. 1997. Landscape characterization of peridomestic risk for Lyme disease using satellite imagery. American Journal of Tropical Medicine and Hygiene 57:687–692.

DiTomaso, J. M. 2000. Invasive weeds in rangelands: species, impacts, and management. Weed Science 48:255–265.

Dixon, J. and B. F. Menezes. 2009. Predictors of mortality and morbidity in *Clostridium difficile* infections. International Journal of Collaborative Research on Internal Medicine and Public Health 1:23–26.

Dizney, L. J., and L. A. Ruedas. 2009. Increased host species diversity and decreased prevalence of Sin Nombre virus. Emerging Infectious Diseases 15:1012–1018.

Dobson, A., I. Cattadori, R. D. Holt, R. S. Ostfeld, F. Keesing, K. Krichbaum, J. R. Rohr, S. E. Perkins, and P. J. Hudson. 2006. Sacred cows and sympathetic squirrels: the importance of biological diversity to human health. PLoS Medicine 3:714–718.

Dolan, M. C., G. O. Maupin, B. S. Schneider, C. Denatale, N. Hamon, C. Cole, N. S. Zeidner, and K. C. Stafford. 2004. Control of immature *Ixodes scapularis* (Acari: Ixodidae) on rodent reservoirs of *Borrelia burgdorferi* in a residential community of southeastern Connecticut. Journal of Medical Entomology 41: 1043–1054.

Donahue, J. G., J. Piesman, and A. Spielman. 1987. Reservoir competence of white-footed mice for Lyme disease spirochetes. American Journal of Tropical Medicine and Hygiene 36:92–96.

Duffy, D. C., S. R. Campbell, D. Clark, C. Dimotta, and S. Gurney. 1994. *Ixodes scapularis* (Acari: Ixodidae) deer tick mesoscale populations in natural areas—effects of deer, area, and location. Journal of Medical Entomology 31:152–158.

Duffy, D. C., R. Downer, and C. Brinkley. 1992. The effectiveness of helmeted guinea fowl in the control of the deer tick, the vector of Lyme disease. Wilson Bulletin 104:342–345.

Edlow, J. A. 2003. Bull's Eye: Unraveling the Medical Mystery of Lyme Disease. Yale University Press, New Haven.

Eisen, R. J., R. S. Lane, C. L. Fritz, and L. Eisen. 2006. Spatial patterns of Lyme disease risk in California based on disease incidence data and modeling of vector-tick exposure. American Journal of Tropical Medicine and Hygiene 75:669–676.

Elkinton, J. S., W. M. Healy, J. P. Buonaccorsi, G. H. Boettner, A. M. Hazzard, H. R. Smith, and A. M. Liebhold. 1996. Interactions among gypsy moths, white-footed mice, and acorns. Ecology 77:2332–2342.

Elton, C. S. 1966. The Pattern of Animal Communities. Wiley, London.

Estrada-Peña, A. 1998. Geostatistics and remote sensing as predictive tools of tick distribution: a cokriging system to estimate *Ixodes scapularis* (Acari: Ixodidae) habitat suitability in the United States and Canada from advanced very high resolution radiometer satellite imagery. Journal of Medical Entomology 35:989–995.

European Commission. 2007. Attitudes of Europeans toward the Issue of Biodiversity—Analytical Report. Flash Eurobarometer no. 219. Gallup Organization. Available: ec.europa.eu/public_opinion/flash/fl_219_en.pdf.

Ezenwa, V. O., M. S. Godsey, R. J. King, and S. C. Guptill. 2006. Avian diversity and West Nile virus: testing associations between biodiversity and infectious disease risk. Proceedings of the Royal Society, Series B, Biological Sciences 273:109–117.

Falco, R. C., and D. Fish. 1988. Prevalence of *Ixodes dammini* near the homes of Lyme disease patients in Westchester County, New York. American Journal of Epidemiology 127:826–830.

Field, H. E., J. S. Mackenzie, and P. Daszak. 2007. Henipaviruses: emerging paramyxoviruses associated with fruit bats. Pages 113–159 *in* Wildlife and Emerging Zoonotic Diseases: The Biology, Circumstances and Consequences of Cross-Species Transmission (J. E. Childs, J. S. Mackenzie, and J. A. Richt, editors). Current Topics in Microbiology and Immunology no. 315. Springer, Berlin.

Fish, D. 1993. Population ecology of *Ixodes dammini*. Pages 25–42 *in* Ecology and Environmental Management of Lyme Disease (H. S. Ginsberg, editor). Rutgers University Press, New Brunswick, N.J.

Fish, D. 1995. Environmental risk and prevention of Lyme disease. American Journal of Medicine 98:S2–S9.

Fish, D., and T. J. Daniels. 1990. The role of medium-sized mammals as reservoirs of *Borrelia burgdorferi* in southern New York. Journal of Wildlife Diseases 26:339–345.

Fish, D., and R. C. Dowler. 1989. Host associations of ticks (Acari: Ixodidae) parasitizing medium-sized mammals in a Lyme disease endemic area of southern New York. Journal of Medical Entomology 26:200–209.

Frank, D. H., D. Fish, and F. H. Moy. 1998. Landscape features associated with Lyme disease risk in a suburban residential environment. Landscape Ecology 13:27–36.

Freimoser, F. M., G. Hu, and R. J. St. Leger. 2005. Variation in gene expression patterns as the insect pathogen *Metarhizium anisopliae* adapts to different host cuticles or nutrient deprivation in vitro. Microbiology-Sgm 151:361–371.

Freimoser, F. M., S. Screen, S. Bagga, G. Hu, and R. J. St. Leger. 2003. Expressed sequence tag (EST) analysis of two subspecies of *Metarhizium anisopliae* reveals a plethora of secreted proteins with potential activity in insect hosts. Microbiology 149:239–247.

Gaskin, A. A., P. Schantz, J. Jackson, A. Birkenheuer, L. Tomlinson, M. Gramiccia, M. Levy, F. Steurer, E. Kollmar, B. C. Hegarty, A. Ahn, and E. B. Breitschwerdt. 2002. Visceral leishmaniasis in a New York foxhound kennel. Journal of Veterinary Internal Medicine 16:34–44.

Gage, K. L., R. S. Ostfeld, and J. G. Olson. 1995. Nonviral vector-borne zoonoses associated with mammals in the United States. Journal of Mammalogy 76:695–715.

Gern, L. 2008. *Borrelia burgdorferi sensu lato,* the agent of Lyme borreliosis: life in the wilds. Parasite 15:244–247.

Giardina, A. R., K. A. Schmidt, E. M. Schauber, and R. S. Ostfeld. 2000. Modeling the role of songbirds and rodents in the ecology of Lyme disease. Canadian Journal of Zoology 78:2184–2197.

Giery, S. T., and R. S. Ostfeld. 2007. The role of lizards in the ecology of Lyme disease in two endemic zones of the northeastern United States. Journal of Parasitology 93:511–517.

Ginsberg, H. S., R. A. Lebrun, K. Heyer, and E. Zhioua. 2002. Potential nontarget effects of *Metarhizium anisopliae* (Deuteromycetes) used for biological control of ticks (Acari: Ixodidae). Environmental Entomology 31:1191–1196.

Glass, G. E., F. P. Amerasinghe, J. M. Morgan, and T. W. Scott. 1994. Predicting *Ixodes scapularis* abundance on white-tailed deer using geographic information systems. American Journal of Tropical Medicine and Hygiene 51:538–544.

Glass, G. E., B. S. Schwartz, J. M. Morgan, D. T. Johnson, P. M. Noy, and E. Israel. 1995. Environmental risk factors for Lyme disease identified with geographic information systems. American Journal of Public Health 85:944–948.

Guan, Y., B. J. Zheng, Y. Q. He, X. L. Liu, Z. X. Zhuang, C. L. Cheung, S. W. Luo, P. H. Li, L. J. Zhang, Y. J. Guan, K. M. Butt, K. L. Wong, K. W. Chan, W. Lim, K. F. Shortridge, K. Y. Yuen, J. S. M. Peiris, and L. L. M. Poon. 2003. Isolation and characterization of viruses related to the SARS coronavirus from animals in Southern China. Science 302:276–278.

Guerra, M., E. Walker, C. Jones, S. Paskewitz, M. R. Cortinas, A. Stancil, L. Beck, M. Bobo, and U. Kitron. 2002. Predicting the risk of Lyme disease: habitat suitability for *Ixodes scapularis* in the north central United States. Emerging Infectious Diseases 8:289–297.

Holt, R. D. 2008. Theoretical perspectives on resource pulses. Ecology 89:671–681.

Hornbostel, V. L., R. S. Ostfeld, E. Zhioua, and M. A. Benjamin. 2004. Sublethal effects of *Metarhizium anisopliae* (Deuteromycetes) on engorged larval, nymphal, and adult *Ixodes scapularis* (Acari: Ixodidae). Journal of Medical Entomology 41:922–929.

Horobik, V., F. Keesing, and R. S. Ostfeld. 2006. Abundance and *Borrelia burgdorferi* infection prevalence of nymphal *Ixodes scapularis* ticks along forest-field edges. EcoHealth 3:262–268.

Hurlbert, S. H. 1984. Pseudoreplication and the design of ecological field experiments. Ecological Monographs 54:187–211.

Jackson, L. E., E. D. Hilborn, and J. C. Thomas. 2006a. Towards landscape design guidelines for reducing Lyme disease risk. International Journal of Epidemiology 35: 315–322.

Jackson, L. E., J. F. Levine, and E. D. Hilborn. 2006b. A comparison of analysis units for associating Lyme disease with forest-edge habitat. Community Ecology 7:189–197.

Johnson, P. T. J., P. J. Lund, R. B. Hartson, and T. P. Yoshino. 2009. Community diversity reduces *Schistosoma mansoni* transmission, host pathology and human infection risk. Proceedings of the Royal Society, Series B, Biological Sciences 276:1657–1663.

Johnson, R. C., G. P. Schmid, F. W. Hyde, A. G. Steigerwalt, and D. J. Brenner. 1984. *Borrelia burgdorferi* sp-nov—etiologic agent of Lyme disease. International Journal of Systematic Bacteriology 34:496–497.

Jones, C. G., R. S. Ostfeld, M. P. Richard, E. M. Schauber, and J. O. Wolff. 1998. Chain reactions linking acorns to gypsy moth outbreaks and Lyme disease risk. Science 279:1023–1026.

Jones, C. J., and U. D. Kitron. 2000. Populations of *Ixodes scapularis* (Acari : Ixodidae) are modulated by drought at a Lyme disease focus in Illinois. Journal of Medical Entomology 37:408–415.

Jordan, R. A., and T. L. Schulze. 2005. Deer browsing and the distribution of *Ixodes scapularis* (Acari: Ixodidae) in central New Jersey forests. Environmental Entomology 34:801–806.

Jordan, R. A., T. L. Schulze, and M. B. Jahn. 2007. Effects of reduced deer density on the abundance of *Ixodes scapularis* (Acari: Ixodidae) and Lyme disease incidence in a northern New Jersey endemic area. Journal of Medical Entomology 44:752–757.

Jouda, F., J. L. Perret, and L. Gern. 2004. *Ixodes ricinus* density, and distribution and prevalence of *Borrelia burgdorferi sensu lato* infection along an altitudinal gradient. Journal of Medical Entomology 41:162–169.

Kan, B., M. Wang, H. Q. Jing, H. F. Xu, X. G. Jiang, M. Y. Yan, W. L. Liang, H. Zheng, K. L. Wan, Q. Y. Liu, B. Y. Cui, Y. M. Xu, E. M. Zhang, H. X. Wang, J. R. Ye, G. H. Li, M. H. Li, Z. G. Cui, X. B. Qi, K. Chen, L. Du, K. Gao, Y. T. Zhao, X. Z. Zou, Y. J. Feng, Y. F. Gao, R. Hai, D. Z. Yu, Y. Guan, and J. G. Xu. 2005. Molecular evolution analysis and geographic investigation of severe acute respiratory syndrome coronavirus-like virus in palm civets at an animal market and on farms. Journal of Virology 79:11892–11900.

Kays, R. W., and D. E. Wilson. 2002. Mammals of North America. Princeton University Press, Princeton, N.J.

Keesing, F., J. Brunner, S. Duerr, M. Killilea, K. LoGiudice, K. Schmidt, H. Vuong, and R. S. Ostfeld. 2009. Hosts as ecological traps for the vector of Lyme disease. Proceedings of the Royal Society, Series B, Biological Sciences 276:3911–3919.

Keesing, F., R. D. Holt, and R. S. Ostfeld. 2006. Effects of species diversity on disease risk. Ecology Letters 9:485–498.

Keirans, J. E., H. J. Hutcheson, L. A. Durden, and J. S. H. Klompen. 1996. *Ixodes scapularis* (Acari: Ixodidae): redescription of all active stages, distribution, hosts, geographical variation, and medical and veterinary importance. Journal of Medical Entomology 33:297–318.

Kennamer, J. E., M. Kennamer, and R. Brenneman. 1992. History. Pages 6–17 *in* The Wild Turkey: Biology and Management (J. G. Dickson, ed.). Stackpole Press, Mechanicsburg, Pennsylvania.

Killilea, M. E., A. Swei, R. S. Lane, C. J. Briggs, and R. S. Ostfeld. 2008. Spatial dynamics of Lyme disease: a review. EcoHealth 5:167–195.

Kilpatrick, A. M., P. Daszak, S. J. Goodman, H. Rogg, L. D. Kramer, V. Cedeno, and A. A. Cunningham. 2006a. Predicting pathogen introduction: West Nile virus spread to Galapagos. Conservation Biology 20:1224–1231.

Kilpatrick, A. M., P. Daszak, M. J. Jones, P. P. Marra, and L. D. Kramer. 2006b. Host heterogeneity dominates West Nile virus transmission. Proceedings of the Royal Society, Series B, Biological Sciences 273:2327–2333.

Kilpatrick, A. M., L. D. Kramer, M. J. Jones, P. P. Marra, P. Daszak, and D. M. Fonseca. 2007. Genetic influences on mosquito feeding behavior and the emergence of zoonotic pathogens. American Journal of Tropical Medicine and Hygiene 77:667–671.

Kitron, U., C. J. Jones, and J. K. Bouseman. 1991. Spatial and temporal dispersion of immature *Ixodes dammini* on *Peromyscus leucopus* in northwestern Illinois. Journal of Parasitology 77:945–949.

Kitron, U., and J. J. Kazmierczak. 1997. Spatial analysis of the distribution of Lyme disease in Wisconsin. American Journal of Epidemiology 145:558–566.

Klingstrom, J., P. Heyman, S. Escutenaire, K. B. Sjolander, F. De Jaegere, H. Henttonen, and A. Lundkvist. 2002. Rodent host specificity of European hantaviruses: evidence of Puumala virus interspecific spillover. Journal of Medical Virology 68:581–588.

Knops, J. M. H., D. Tilman, N. M. Haddad, S. Naeem, C. E. Mitchell, J. Haarstad, M. E. Ritchie, K. M. Howe, P. B. Reich, E. Siemann, and J. Groth. 1999. Effects of plant species richness on invasion dynamics, disease outbreaks, insect abundances and diversity. Ecology Letters 2:286–293.

Komar, N., S. Langevin, S. Hinten, N. Nemeth, E. Edwards, D. Hettler, B. Davis, R. Bowen, and M. Bunning. 2003. Experimental infection of North American birds with the New York 1999 strain of West Nile virus. Emerging Infectious Diseases 9:311–322.

Komar, O., M. B. Robbins, G. G. Contreras, B. W. Benz, K. Klenk, B. J. Blitvich, N. L. Marlenee, K. L. Burkhalter, S. Beckett, G. Gonzalvez, C. J. Pena, A. T. Peterson, and N. Komar. 2005. West Nile virus survey of birds and mosquitoes in the Dominican Republic. Vector-Borne and Zoonotic Diseases 5:120–126.

Krasnov, B. R., D. Mouillot, I. S. Khokhlova, G. I. Shenbrot, and R. Poulin. 2008. Scale-invariance of niche breadth in fleas parasitic on small mammals. Ecography 31:630–635.

Krebs, C. J. 1989. Ecological Methodology. Harper Collins, New York.

Kuenzi, A. J., R. J. Douglass, D. White, C. W. Bond, and J. N. Mills. 2001. Antibody to Sin Nombre virus in rodents associated with peridomestic habitats in west central Montana. American Journal of Tropical Medicine and Hygiene 64:137–146.

Labuda, M., L. D. Jones, T. Williams, V. Danielova, and P. A. Nuttall. 1993. Efficient transmission of tick-borne encephalitis virus between cofeeding ticks. Journal of Medical Entomology 30:295–299.

LaDeau, S. L., A. M. Kilpatrick, and P. P. Marra. 2007. West Nile virus emergence and large-scale declines of North American bird populations. Nature 447:710-U713.

LaDeau, S. L., P. P. Marra, A. M. Kilpatrick, and C. A. Calder. 2008. West Nile virus revisited: consequences for North American ecology. Bioscience 58:937–946.

Lane, R. S., J. Piesman, and W. Burgdorfer. 1991. Lyme borreliosis—relation of its causative agent to its vectors and hosts in North America and Europe. Annual Review of Entomology 36:587–609.

Lane, R. S., and G. B. Quistad. 1998. Borreliacidal factor in the blood of the western fence lizard (*Sceloporus occidentalis*). Journal of Parasitology 84:29–34.

LaRocca, T. J., and J. L. Benach. 2008. The important and diverse roles of antibodies in the host response to *Borrelia* infections. Pages 63–103 *in* Specialization and Complementation of Humoral Immune Responses to Infection (T. Manser, editor). Current Topics in Microbiology and Immunology no. 319. Springer, Berlin.

Lawley, T. D., S. Clare, A. W. Walker, D. Goulding, R. A. Stabler, N. Croucher, P. Mastroeni, P. Scott, C. Raisen, L. Mottram, N. F. Fairweather, B. W. Wren, J. Parkhill, and G. Dougan. 2009. Antibiotic treatment of *Clostridium difficile* carrier mice triggers a supershedder state, spore-mediated transmission, and severe disease in immunocompromised hosts. Infection and Immunity 77:3661–3669.

Levine, J. F., M. L. Wilson, and A. Spielman. 1985. Mice as reservoirs of the Lyme disease spirochete. American Journal of Tropical Medicine and Hygiene 34:355–360.

Lewellen, R. H., and S. H. Vessey. 1998. The effect of density dependence and weather on population size of a polyvoltine species. Ecological Monographs 68:571–594.

Li, W. D., Z. L. Shi, M. Yu, W. Z. Ren, C. Smith, J. H. Epstein, H. Z. Wang, G. Crameri, Z. H. Hu, H. J. Zhang, J. H. Zhang, J. McEachern, H. Field, P. Daszak, B. T. Eaton, S. Y. Zhang, and L. F. Wang. 2005. Bats are natural reservoirs of SARS-like coronaviruses. Science 310:676–679.

Lidicker, W. Z., Jr. 1991. In defense of a multifactor perspective in population ecology. Journal of Mammalogy 72:631–635.

Lindsay, L. R., I. K. Barker, G. A. Surgeoner, S. A. McEwen, T. J. Gillespie, and E. M. Addison. 1998. Survival and development of the different life stages of *Ixodes scapularis* (Acari: Ixodidae) held within four habitats on Long Point, Ontario, Canada. Journal of Medical Entomology 35:189–199.

Lindsay, L. R., I. K. Barker, G. A. Surgeoner, S. A. McEwen, T. J. Gillespie, and J. T. Robinson. 1995. Survival and development of *Ixodes scapularis* (Acari: Ixodidae) under various climatic conditions in Ontario, Canada. Journal of Medical Entomology 32:143–152.

LoGiudice, K., S. T. K. Duerr, M. J. Newhouse, K. A. Schmidt, M. E. Killilea, and R. S. Ostfeld. 2008. Impact of host community composition on Lyme disease risk. Ecology 89:2841–2849.

LoGiudice, K., R. S. Ostfeld, K. A. Schmidt, and F. Keesing. 2003. The ecology of infectious disease: effects of host diversity and community composition on Lyme disease risk. Proceedings of the National Academy of Sciences of the United States of America 100:567–571.

Loss, S. R., G. L. Hamer, E. D. Walker, M. O. Ruiz, T. L. Goldberg, U. D. Kitron, and J. D. Brawn. 2009. Avian host community structure and prevalence of West Nile virus in Chicago, Illinois. Oecologia 159:415–424.

Lubelczyk, C. B., S. P. Elias, P. W. Rand, M. S. Holman, E. H. Lacombe, and R. P. Smith. 2004. Habitat associations of *Ixodes scapularis* (Acari: Ixodidae) in Maine. Environmental Entomology 33:900–906.

MacArthur, R. H., and E. O. Wilson. 1967. The Theory of Island Biogeography. Princeton University Press, Princeton, N.J.

Macdonald, G. 1957. The Epidemiology and Control of Malaria. Oxford University Press, London.

Madhav, N. K., J. S. Brownstein, J. I. Tsao, and D. Fish. 2004. A dispersal model for the range expansion of blacklegged tick (Acari: Ixodidae). Journal of Medical Entomology 41:842–852.

Magnarelli, L. A., J. F., Anderson, W. Burgdorfer, and W. A. Chappell. 1984. Parasitism by *Ixodes dammini* (Acari: Ixodidae) and antibodies to spirochetes in mammals at Lyme disease foci in Connecticut, USA. Journal of Medical Entomology 21:52–57.

Main, A. J., A. B. Carey, M. G. Carey, and R. H. Goodwin. 1982. Immature *Ixodes dammini* (Acari: Ixodidae) on small animals in Connecticut, USA. Journal of Medical Entomology 19:655–664.

Main, A. J., H. E. Sprance, K. O. Kloter, and S. E. Brown. 1981. *Ixodes dammini* (Acari: Ixodidae) on white-tailed deer (*Odocoileus virginianus*) in Connecticut. Journal of Medical Entomology 18:487–492.

Marra, M. A., S. J. M. Jones, C. R. Astell, R. A. Holt, A. Brooks-Wilson, Y. S. N. Butterfield, J. Khattra, J. K. Asano, S. A. Barber, S. Y. Chan, A. Cloutier, S. M. Coughlin, D. Freeman, N. Girn, O. L. Griffith, S. R. Leach, M. Mayo, H. McDonald, S. B. Montgomery, P. K. Pandoh, A. S. Petrescu, A. G. Robertson, J. E. Schein, A. Siddiqui, D. E. Smailus, J. E. Stott, G. S. Yang, F. Plummer, A., Andonov, H. Artsob, N. Bastien, K. Bernard, T. F. Booth, D. Bowness, M. Czub, M. Drebot, L. Fernando, R. Flick, M. Garbutt, M. Gray, A. Grolla, S. Jones, H. Feldmann, A. Meyers, A. Kabani, Y. Li, S. Normand, U. Stroher, G. A. Tipples, S. Tyler, R. Vogrig, D. Ward, B. Watson, R. C. Brunham, M. Krajden, M. Petric, D. M. Skowronski, C. Upton, and R. L. Roper. 2003. The genome sequence of the SARS-associated coronavirus. Science 300:1399–1404.

Marra, P. P., S. Griffing, C. Caffrey, A. M. Kilpatrick, R. McLean, C. Brand, E. Saito, A. P. Dupuis, L. Kramer, and R. Novak. 2004. West Nile virus and wildlife. Bioscience 54:393–402.

Martin, L. B. 2009. Stress and immunity in wild vertebrates: timing is everything. General and Comparative Endocrinology 163:70–76.

Martin, L. B., Z. M. Weil, and R. J. Nelson. 2008. Seasonal changes in vertebrate immune activity: mediation by physiological trade-offs. Philosophical Transactions of the Royal Society, Series B, Biological Sciences 363:321–339.

Mather, T. N. 1993. The dynamics of spirochete transmission between ticks and verte-brates. Pages 43–60 *in* Ecology and Environmental Management of Lyme Disease (H. S. Ginsberg, editor). Rutgers University Press, New Brunswick, N.J.

Mather, T. N., D. C. Duffy, and S. R. Campbell. 1993. An unexpected result from burning vegetation to reduce Lyme disease transmission risks. Journal of Medical Entomology 30:642–645.

Mather, T. N., J. M. C. Ribeiro, and A. Spielman. 1987. Lyme disease and babesiosis acari-cide focused on potentially infected ticks. American Journal of Tropical Medicine and Hygiene 36:609–614.

Mather, T. N., S. R. Telford, S. I. Moore, and A. Spielman. 1990. *Borrelia burgdorferi* and *Babesia microti*—efficiency of transmission from reservoirs to vector ticks (*Ixodes dammini*). Experimental Parasitology 70:55–61.

Mather, T. N., M. L. Wilson, S. I. Moore, J. M. C. Ribeiro, and A. Spielman. 1989. Com-paring the relative potential of rodents as reservoirs of the Lyme disease spirochete (*Borrelia burgdorferi*). American Journal of Epidemiology 130:143–150.

Maupin, G. O., D. Fish, J. Zultowsky, E. G. Campos, and J. Piesman. 1991. Landscape ecology of Lyme disease in a residential area of Westchester County, New York. American Journal of Epidemiology 133:1105–1113.

McCabe, G. J., and J. E. Bunnell. 2004. Precipitation and the occurrence of Lyme disease in the northeastern United States. Vector-Borne and Zoonotic Diseases 4:143–148.

McEnroe, W. D. 1977. Restriction of species range of *Ixodes scapularis* (Say) in Massachu-setts by fall and winter temperature. Acarologia 18:618–625.

McShea, W. J., S. L. Monfort, S. Hakim, J. Kirkpatrick, I. Liu, J. W. Turner, L. Chassy, and L. Munson. 1997. The effect of immunocontraception on the behavior and reproduc-tion of white-tailed deer. Journal of Wildlife Management 61:560–569.

Mills, J. N., J. M. Johnson, T. G. Ksiazek, B. A. Ellis, P. E. Rollin, T. L. Yates, M. O. Minn, M. R. Johnson, M. L. Campbell, J. Miyashiro, M. Patrick, M. Zyzak, D. Lavender, M. G. Novak, K. Schmidt, C. J. Peters, and J. E. Childs. 1998. A survey of hantavirus anti-body in small-mammal populations in selected United States National Parks. Ameri-can Journal of Tropical Medicine and Hygiene 58:525–532.

Mills, J. N., T. G. Ksiazek, B. A. Ellis, P. E. Rollin, S. T. Nichol, T. L. Yates, W. L. Gannon, C. E. Levy, D. M. Engelthaler, T. Davis, D. T. Tanda, J. W. Frampton, C. R. Nichols, C. J. Peters, and J. E. Childs. 1997. Patterns of association with host and habitat: antibody reactive with Sin Nombre virus in small mammals in the major biotic communities of the southwestern United States. American Journal of Tropical Medicine and Hygiene 56:273–284.

Mitchell, C. E., P. B. Reich, D. Tilman, and J. V. Groth. 2003. Effects of elevated CO_2, nitro-gen deposition, and decreased species diversity on foliar fungal plant disease. Global Change Biology 9:438–451.

Mitchell, C. E., D. Tilman, and J. V. Groth. 2002. Effects of grassland plant species diversity, abundance, and composition on foliar fungal disease. Ecology 83:1713–1726.

Mount, G. A., D. G. Haile, and E. Daniels. 1997. Simulation of blacklegged tick (Acari: Ixodidae) population dynamics and transmission of *Borrelia burgdorferi*. Journal of Medical Entomology 34:461–484.

Muller-Doblies, U. U., S. S. Maxwell, V. D. Boppana, M. A. Mihalyo, S. J. Mcsorley, A. T. Vella, A. J. Adler, and S. K. Wikel. 2007. Feeding by the tick, *Ixodes scapularis,* causes CD4(+) T cells responding to cognate antigen to develop the capacity to express IL-4. Parasite Immunology 29:485–499.

Myers, P., R. Espinosa, C. S. Parr, T. Jones, G. S. Hammond, and T. A. Dewey. 2006. The Animal Diversity Web (online). Accessed January 02, 2010 at http://animaldiversity.org.

Naeem, S., D. E. Bunker, A. Hector, M. Loreau, and C. Perrings, editors. 2009. Biodiversity, Ecosystem Functioning, and Human Wellbeing—An Ecological and Economic Perspective. Oxford University Press, New York.

Normile, D., and Y. M. Ding. 2003. Infectious diseases—civets back on China's menu. Science 301:1031–1031.

Norris, D. E., J. S. H. Klompen, J. E. Keirans, and W. C. Black. 1996. Population genetics of *Ixodes scapularis* (Acari: Ixodidae) based on mitochondrial 16S and 12S genes. Journal of Medical Entomology 33:78–89.

Nupp, T. E., and R. K. Swihart. 1998. Effects of forest fragmentation on population attributes of white-footed mice and eastern chipmunks. Journal of Mammalogy 79: 1234–1243.

Ogden, N. H., M. Bigras-Poulin, K. Hanincova, A. Maarouf, C. J. O'Callaghan, and K. Kurtenbach. 2008a. Projected effects of climate change on tick phenology and fitness of pathogens transmitted by the North American tick *Ixodes scapularis.* Journal of Theoretical Biology 254:621–632.

Ogden, N. H., M. Bigras-Poulin, C. J. O'Callaghan, I. K. Barker, L. R. Lindsay, A. Maarouf, K. E. Smoyer-Tomic, D. Waltner-Toews, and D. Charron. 2005. A dynamic population model to investigate effects of climate on geographic range and seasonality of the tick *Ixodes scapularis.* International Journal for Parasitology 35:375–389.

Ogden, N. H., L. R. Lindsay, G. Beauchamp, D. Charron, A. Maarouf, C. J. O'Callaghan, D. Waltner-Toews, and I. K. Barker. 2004. Investigation of relationships between temperature and developmental rates of tick *Ixodes scapularis* (Acari: Ixodidae) in the laboratory and field. Journal of Medical Entomology 41:622–633.

Ogden, N. H., L. R. Lindsay, M. Morshed, P. N. Sockett, and H. Artsob. 2009. The emergence of Lyme disease in Canada. Canadian Medical Association Journal 180: 1221–1224.

Ogden, N. H., A. Maarouf, I. K. Barker, M. Bigras-Poulin, L. R. Lindsay, M. G. Morshed, C. J. O'Callaghan, F. Ramay, D. Waltner-Toews, and D. F. Charron. 2006. Climate change and the potential for range expansion of the Lyme disease vector *Ixodes scapularis* in Canada. International Journal for Parasitology 36:63–70.

Ogden, N. H., L. St-Onge, I. K. Barker, S. Brazeau, M. Bigras-Poulin, D. F. Charron, C. M. Francis, A. Heagy, L. R. Lindsay, A. Maarouf, P. Michel, F. Milord, C. J. O'Callaghan, L. Trudel, and R. A. Thompson. 2008b. Risk maps for range expansion of the Lyme disease vector, *Ixodes scapularis,* in Canada now and with climate change. International Journal of Health Geographics 7:24.

Oliver, J. H., M. R. Owsley, H. J. Hutcheson, A. M. James, C. S. Chen, W. S. Irby, E. M. Dotson, and D. K. McLain. 1993. Conspecificity of the ticks *Ixodes scapularis* and *Ixodes dammini* (Acari: Ixodidae). Journal of Medical Entomology 30:54–63.

Orloski, K. A., G. L. Campbell, C. A. Genese, J. W. Beckley, M. E. Schriefer, K. C. Spitalny, and D. T. Dennis. 1998. Emergence of Lyme disease in Hunterdon County, New Jersey, 1993: a case-control study of risk factors and evaluation of reporting patterns. American Journal of Epidemiology 147:391–397.

Ostfeld, R.S. 2009. Biodiversity loss and the rise of zoonotic pathogens. Clinical Microbiology and Infection 15 (Suppl 1): 40–43.

Ostfeld, R. S., C. D. Canham, K. Oggenfuss, R. J. Winchcombe, and F. Keesing. 2006a. Climate, deer, rodents, and acorns as determinants of variation in Lyme disease risk. PLoS Biology 4:1058–1068.

Ostfeld, R. S., O. M. Cepeda, K. R. Hazler, and M. C. Miller. 1995. Ecology of Lyme disease habitat associations of ticks (*Ixodes scapularis*) in a rural landscape. Ecological Applications 5:353–361.

Ostfeld, R. S., K. R. Hazler, and O. M. Cepeda. 1996a. Temporal and spatial dynamics of *Ixodes scapularis* (Acari: Ixodidae) in a rural landscape. Journal of Medical Entomology 33:90–95.

Ostfeld, R. S., and R. D. Holt. 2004. Are predators good for your health? Evaluating evidence for top-down regulation of zoonotic disease reservoirs. Frontiers in Ecology and the Environment 2:13–20.

Ostfeld, R. S., C. G. Jones, and J. O. Wolff. 1996b. Of mice and mast. Bioscience 46:323–330.

Ostfeld, R., and F. Keesing. 2000a. The function of biodiversity in the ecology of vector-borne zoonotic diseases. Canadian Journal of Zoology 78:2061–2078.

Ostfeld, R. S., and F. Keesing. 2000b. Biodiversity and disease risk: the case of Lyme disease. Conservation Biology 14:722–728.

Ostfeld, R. S., and F. Keesing. 2000c. Pulsed resources and community dynamics of consumers in terrestrial ecosystems. Trends in Ecology and Evolution 15:232–237.

Ostfeld, R., F. Keesing, and K. LoGiudice. 2006b. Community ecology meets epidemiology: the case of Lyme disease. Pages 28–40 *in* Disease Ecology: Community Structure and Pathogen Dynamics (S. Collinge and C. Ray, editors). Oxford University Press, New York.

Ostfeld, R. S., and D. Lewis. 1999. Experimental studies of interactions between wild turkeys and blacklegged ticks. Journal of Vector Ecology 24:182–186.

Ostfeld, R. S., and K. LoGiudice. 2003. Community disassembly, biodiversity loss, and the erosion of an ecosystem service. Ecology 84:1421–1427.

Ostfeld, R. S., A. Price, V. L. Hornbostel, M. A. Benjamin, and F. Keesing. 2006c. Controlling ticks and tick-borne zoonoses with biological and chemical agents. Bioscience 56:383–394.

Ostfeld, R. S., P. Roy, W. Haumaier, L. Canter, F. Keesing, and E. D. Rowton. 2004. Sand fly (*Lutzomyia vexator*) (Diptera: Psychodidae) populations in upstate New York: abundance, microhabitat, and phenology. Journal of Medical Entomology 41:774–778.

Ostfeld, R. S., E. M. Schauber, C. D. Canham, F. Keesing, C. G. Jones, and J. O. Wolff. 2001. Effects of acorn production and mouse abundance on abundance and *Borrelia burgdorferi* infection prevalence of nymphal *Ixodes scapularis*. Vector-Borne and Zoonotic Diseases 1:55–64.

Patrican, L. A. 1997. Absence of Lyme disease spirochetes in larval progeny of naturally infected *Ixodes scapularis* (Acari: Ixodidae) fed on dogs. Journal of Medical Entomology 34:52–55.

Pearson, D. E., and R. M. Callaway. 2006. Biological control agents elevate hantavirus by subsidizing deer mouse populations. Ecology Letters 9:443–450.

Perkins, S. E., I. M. Cattadori, V. Tagliapietra, A. P. Rizzoli, and P. J. Hudson. 2006. Localized deer absence leads to tick amplification. Ecology 87:1981–1986.

Piesman, J. 1987. Emerging tick-borne diseases in temperate climates. Parasitology Today 3:197–199.

Piesman, J. 2002. Ecology of *Borrelia burgdorferi sensu lato* in North America. Page 347 *in* Lyme Borreliosis—Biology, Epidemiology and Control (J. S. Gray, O. Kahl, R. S. Lane, and G. Stanek, editors). CABI Publishing, New York.

Piesman, J., J. G. Donahue, T. N. Mather, and A. Spielman. 1986. Transovarially acquired Lyme disease spirochetes (*Borrelia burgdorferi*) in field-collected larval *Ixodes dammini* (Acari: Ixodidae). Journal of Medical Entomology 23:219–219.

Piesman, J., and A. Spielman. 1979. Host associations and seasonal abundance of immature *Ixodes dammini* (Acarina: Ixodidae) in southeastern Massachusetts. Annals of the Entomological Society of America 72:829–832.

Piesman, J., A. Spielman, P. Etkind, T. K. Ruebush, and D. D. Juranek. 1979. Role of deer in the epizootiology of *Babesia microti* in Massachusetts, USA. Journal of Medical Entomology 15:537–540.

Plowright, R. K., H. E. Field, C. Smith, A. Divljan, C. Palmer, G. Tabor, P. Daszak, and J. E. Foley. 2008. Reproduction and nutritional stress are risk factors for Hendra virus infection in little red flying foxes (*Pteropus scapulatus*). Proceedings of the Royal Society, Series B, Biological Sciences 275:861–869.

Poland, G. A. 2001. Prevention of Lyme disease: a review of the evidence. Mayo Clinic Proceedings 76:713–724.

Pool, R. 1991. Science's top 20 greatest hits. Science 251:267.

Pound, J. M., J. A. Miller, and J. E. George. 2000. Efficacy of amitraz applied to white-tailed deer by the "4-poster" topical treatment device in controlling free-living lone star ticks (Acari: Ixodidae). Journal of Medical Entomology 37:878–884.

Power, A. G., and C. E. Mitchell. 2004. Pathogen spillover in disease epidemics. American Naturalist 164:S79–S89.

Primack, R. B. 2006. Essentials of Conservation Biology. Sinauer Associates, Sunderland, Mass.

Rand, P. W., C. Lubelczyk, M. S. Holman, E. H. Lacombe, and R. P. Smith. 2004. Abundance of *Ixodes scapularis* (Acari: Ixodidae) after the complete removal of deer from an isolated offshore island, endemic for Lyme disease. Journal of Medical Entomology 41:779–784.

Rand, P. W., C. Lubelczyk, G. R. Lavigne, S. Elias, M. S. Holman, E. H. Lacombe, and R. P. Smith. 2003. Deer density and the abundance of *Ixodes scapularis* (Acari: Ixodidae). Journal of Medical Entomology 40:179–184.

Randolph, S. E. 2004. Tick ecology: processes and patterns behind the epidemiological risk posed by ixodid ticks as vectors. Parasitology 129:S37–S65.

Randolph, S. E., and K. Storey. 1999. Impact of microclimate on immature tick-rodent host interactions (Acari: Ixodidae): implications for parasite transmission. Journal of Medical Entomology 36:741–748.

Ribeiro, J. M. C., F. Alarcon-Chaidez, I. M. B. Francischetti, B. J. Mans, T. N. Mather, J. G. Valenzuela, and S. K. Wikel. 2006. An annotated catalog of salivary gland transcripts from *Ixodes scapularis* ticks. Insect Biochemistry and Molecular Biology 36:111–129.

Richter, D., A. Spielman, N. Komar, and F. R. Matuschka. 2000. Competence of American robins as reservoir hosts for Lyme disease spirochetes. Emerging Infectious Diseases 6:133–138.

Rodgers, S. E., and T. N. Mather. 2006. Evaluating satellite sensor-derived indices for Lyme disease risk prediction. Journal of Medical Entomology 43:337–343.

Rodgers, S. E., C. P. Zolnik, and T. N. Mather. 2007. Duration of exposure to suboptimal atmospheric moisture affects nymphal blacklegged tick survival. Journal of Medical Entomology 44:372–375.

Rosenblatt, D. L., E. J. Heske, S. L. Nelson, D. M. Barber, M. A. Miller, and B. MacAllister. 1999. Forest fragments in East-central Illinois: islands or habitat patches for mammals? American Midland Naturalist 141:115–123.

Roscher, C., J. Schumacher, O. Foitzik, and E. D. Schultze. 2007. Resistance to rust fungi in *Lolium perenne* depends on within-species variation and performance of the host species in grasslands of different plant diversity. Oecologia 153:173–183.

Rota, P. A., M. S. Oberste, S. S. Monroe, W. A. Nix, R. Campagnoli, J. P. Icenogle, S. Penaranda, B. Bankamp, K. Maher, M. H. Chen, S. X. Tong, A. Tamin, L. Lowe, M. Frace, J. L. DeRisi, Q. Chen, D. Wang, D. D. Erdman, T. C. T. Peret, C. Burns, T. G. Ksiazek, P. E. Rollin, S. Sanchez, S. Liffick, B. Holloway, J. Limor, K. McCaustland, M. Olsen-Rasmussen, R. Fouchier, S. Gunther, A. D. M. E. Osterhaus, C. Drosten, M. A. Pallansch, L. J., Anderson, and W. J. Bellini. 2003. Characterization of a novel coronavirus associated with severe acute respiratory syndrome. Science 300:1394–1399.

Ruedas, L. A., J. Salazar-Bravo, D. S. Tinnin, B. Armien, L. Caceres, A. Garcia, M. A. Diaz, F. Gracia, G. Suzan, C. J. Peters, T. L. Yates, and J. N. Mills. 2004. Community ecology of small mammal populations in Panama following an outbreak of Hantavirus pulmonary syndrome. Journal of Vector Ecology 29:177–191.

Samish, M., and I. Glazer. 2001. Entomopathogenic nematodes for the biocontrol of ticks. Trends in Parasitology 17:368–371.

Saul, A. 2003. Zooprophylaxis or zoopotentiation: the outcome of introducing animals on vector transmission is highly dependent on the mosquito mortality while searching. Malaria Journal 2:23.

Sauvage, F., M. Langlais, and D. Pontier. 2007. Predicting the emergence of human hantavirus disease using a combination of viral dynamics and rodent demographic patterns. Epidemiology and Infection 135:46–56.

Schauber, E. M., R. S. Ostfeld, and A. S. Evans. 2005. What is the best predictor of annual Lyme disease incidence: weather, mice, or acorns? Ecological Applications 15: 575–586.

Schmidt, K. A. 2003. Linking frequencies of acorn masting in temperate forests to long-term population growth rates in a songbird: the veery (*Catharus fuscescens*). Oikos 103:548–558.

Schmidt, K. A., and R. S. Ostfeld. 2001. Biodiversity and the dilution effect in disease ecology. Ecology 82:609–619.

Schmidt, K. A., and R. S. Ostfeld. 2003. Songbird populations in fluctuating environments: predator responses to pulsed resources. Ecology 84:406–415.

Schmidt, K. A., and R. S. Ostfeld. 2008. Numerical and behavioral effects within a pulse-driven system: consequences for shared prey. Ecology 89:635–646.

Schulze, T. L., R. A. Jordan, M. C. Dolan, G. Dietrich, S. P. Healy, and J. Piesman. 2008a. Ability of 4-poster passive topical treatment devices for deer to sustain low population levels of *Ixodes scapularis* (Acari: Ixodidae) after integrated tick management in a residential landscape. Journal of Medical Entomology 45:899–904.

Schulze, T. L., R. A. Jordan, and R. W. Hung. 2001. Potential effects of animal activity on the spatial distribution of *Ixodes scapularis* and *Amblyomma americanum* (Acari: Ixodidae). Environmental Entomology 30:568–577.

Schulze, T. L., R. A. Jordan, C. J. Schulze, and S. P. Healy. 2008b. Suppression of Ixodes scapularis (Acari: Ixodidae) following annual habitat-targeted acaricide applications against fall populations of adults. Journal of the American Mosquito Control Association 24:566–570.

Schulze, T. L., R. A. Jordan, C. J. Schulze, S. P. Healy, M. B. Jahn, and J. Piesman. 2007. Integrated use of 4-poster passive topical treatment devices for deer, targeted acaricide applications, and maxforce TMS bait boxes to rapidly suppress populations of *Ixodes scapularis* (Acari: Ixodidae) in a residential landscape. Journal of Medical Entomology 44:830–839.

Service, M. W. 1991. Agricultural development and arthropod-borne diseases—a review. Revista De Saude Publica 25:165–178.

Shaw, M. T., F. Keesing, R. McGrail, and R. S. Ostfeld. 2003. Factors influencing the distribution of larval blacklegged ticks on rodent hosts. American Journal of Tropical Medicine and Hygiene 68:447–452.

Shi, Z. L., and Z. H. Hu. 2008. A review of studies on animal reservoirs of the SARS coronavirus. Virus Research 133:74–87.

Slajchert, T., U. D. Kitron, C. J. Jones, and A. Mannelli. 1997. Role of the eastern chipmunk (*Tamias striatus*) in the epizootiology of Lyme borreliosis in northwestern Illinois, USA. Journal of Wildlife Diseases 33:40–46.

Smith, H. R. 1985. Wildlife and the gypsy moth. Wildlife Society Bulletin 13:166–174.

Snall, T., R. B. O'Hara, C. Ray, and S. K. Collinge. 2008. Climate-driven spatial dynamics of plague among prairie dog colonies. American Naturalist 171:238–248.

Solberg, V. B., J. A. Miller, T. Hadfield, R. Burge, J. M. Schech, and J. M. Pound. 2003. Control of *Ixodes scapularis* (Acari: Ixodidae) with topical self-application of permethrin by white-tailed deer inhabiting NASA, Beltsville, Maryland. Journal of Vector Ecology 28:117–134.

Sonenshine, D. E. 1993. Biology of Ticks. Oxford University Press, New York.

Spielman, A. 1976. Human babesiosis on Nantucket Island—transmission by nymphal *Ixodes* ticks. American Journal of Tropical Medicine and Hygiene 25:784–787.

Spielman, A., C. M. Clifford, J. Piesman, and M. D. Corwin. 1979. Human babesiosis on Nantucket Island, USA—description of the vector, *Ixodes dammini*, n-sp (Acarina: Ixodidae). Journal of Medical Entomology 15:218–234.

Spielman, A., M. L. Wilson, J. F. Levine, and J. Piesman. 1985. Ecology of *Ixodes dammini*-borne human babesiosis and Lyme disease. Annual Review of Entomology 30:439–460.

Stafford, K. C. 1992. Oviposition and larval dispersal of Ixodes dammini (Acari: Ixodidae). Journal of Medical Entomology 29:129–132.

Stafford, K. C. 1993. Reduced abundance of *Ixodes scapularis* (Acari: Ixodidae) with exclusion of deer by electric fencing. Journal of Medical Entomology 30:986–996.

Stafford, K. C. 1994. Survival of immature *Ixodes scapularis* (Acari: Ixodidae) at different relative humidities. Journal of Medical Entomology 31:310–314.

Stafford, K. C., A. J. Denicola, and H. J. Kilpatrick. 2003. Reduced abundance of *Ixodes scapularis* (Acari : Ixodidae) and the tick parasitoid *Ixodiphagus hookeri* (Hymenoptera: Encyrtidae) with reduction of white-tailed deer. Journal of Medical Entomology 40:642–652.

Stafford, K. C., and L. A. Magnarelli. 1993. Spatial and temporal patterns of *Ixodes scapularis* (Acari: Ixodidae) in southeastern Connecticut. Journal of Medical Entomology 30:762–771.

Stafford, K. C., J. S. Ward, and L. A. Magnarelli. 1998. Impact of controlled burns on the abundance of *Ixodes scapularis* (Acari: Ixodidae). Journal of Medical Entomology 35:510–513.

Stanek, G., F. Strle, J. S. Gray, and G. P. Wormser. 2002. History and characteristics of Lyme borreliosis. Page 347 *in* Lyme Borreliosis—Biology, Epidemiology and Control (J. S. Gray, O. Kahl, R. S. Lane, and G. Stanek, editors). CABI Publishing, New York.

Stenseth, N. C., N. I. Samia, H. Viljugrein, K. L. Kausrud, M. Begon, S. Davis, H. Leirs, V. M. Dubyanskiy, J. Esper, V. S. Ageyev, N. L. Klassovskiy, S. B. Pole, and K. S. Chan. 2006. Plague dynamics are driven by climate variation. Proceedings of the National Academy of Sciences of the United States of America 103:13110–13115.

Subak, S. 2003. Effects of climate on variability in Lyme disease incidence in the northeastern United States. American Journal of Epidemiology 157:531–538.

Suzan, G., E. Marce, J. T. Giermakowski, J. Mills, G. Ceballos, R. Ostfeld, B. Armien, J. Pascale, and T. L. Yates. 2009. Experimental evidence for reduced rodent diversity causing increased hantavirus prevalence. PLoS ONE 4:e5461.

Swaddle, J. P., and S. E. Calos. 2008. Increased avian diversity is associated with lower incidence of human West Nile infection: observation of the dilution effect. PLoS ONE 3:e2488.

Taylor, L. H., S. M. Latham, and M. E. J. Woolhouse. 2001. Risk factors for human disease emergence. Philosophical Transactions of the Royal Society of London Series, Series B, Biological Sciences 356:983–989.

Telford, S. R. III, T. N. Mather, G. H. Adler, and A. Spielman. 1990. Short-tailed shrews as reservoirs of the agents of Lyme disease and human babesiosis. Journal of Parasitology 76:681–683.

Telford, S. R. III, T. N. Mather, S. I. Moore, M. L. Wilson, and A. Spielman. 1988. Incompetence of deer as reservoirs of the Lyme disease spirochete. American Journal of Tropical Medicine and Hygiene 39:105–109.

Tersago, K., A. Schreurs, C. Linard, R. Verhagen, S. Van Dongen, and H. Leirs. 2008. Population, environmental, and community effects on local bank vole (*Myodes glareolus*) Puumala virus infection in an area with low human incidence. Vector-Borne and Zoonotic Diseases 8:235–244.

Thanassi, W. T., and R. T. Schoen. 2000. The Lyme disease vaccine: conception, development, and implementation. Annals of Internal Medicine 132:661–668.

Tsao, J., A. Barbour, C. J. Luke, E. Fikrig, and D. Fish. 2001. OspA immunization decreases transmission of *Borrelia burgdorferi* spirochetes from infected *Peromyscus leucopus* mice to larval *Ixodes scapularis* ticks. Vector-Borne and Zoonotic Diseases 1:65–74.

Tsao, J., J. T. Wootton, J. Bunikis, M. G. Luna, D. Fish, and A. Barbour. 2004. An ecological approach to preventing human infection: vaccinating wild mouse reservoirs intervenes in the Lyme disease cycle. Proceedings of the National Academy of Sciences of the United States of America 101:18159–18164.

Tuininga, A. R., J. L. Miller, S. U. Morath, T. J. Daniels, R. C. Falco, M. Marchese, S. Sahabi, D. Rosa, and K. C. Stafford. 2009. Isolation of entomopathogenic fungi from soils and *Ixodes scapularis* (Acari: Ixodidae) ticks: prevalence and methods. Journal of Medical Entomology 46:557–565.

Turner, W. R., K. Brandon, T. M. Brooks, R. Costanza, G. A. B. da Fonseca, and R. Portela. 2007. Global conservation of biodiversity and ecosystem services. Bioscience 57: 868–873.

Vail, S. G., and G. Smith. 2002. Vertical movement and posture of blacklegged tick (Acari: Ixodidae) nymphs as a function of temperature and relative humidity in laboratory experiments. Journal of Medical Entomology 39:842–846.

Van Buskirk, J., and R. S. Ostfeld. 1995. Controlling Lyme disease by modifying the density and species composition of tick hosts. Ecological Applications 5:1133–1140.

Wallis, R. C., S. E. Brown, K. O. Kloter, and A. J. Main. 1978. Erythema chronicum migrans and Lyme arthritis—field-study of ticks. American Journal of Epidemiology 108: 322–327.

Weintraub, P. 2008. Cure Unknown—Inside the Lyme Epidemic. St. Martin's Press, New York.

Wesson, D. M., D. K. Mclain, J. H. Oliver, J. Piesman, and F. H. Collins. 1993. Investigation of the validity of species status of *Ixodes dammini* (Acari: Ixodidae) using rDNA. Proceedings of the National Academy of Sciences of the United States of America 90:10221–10225.

Wilson, M. L., G. H. Adler, and A. Spielman. 1985. Correlation between abundance of deer and that of the deer tick, *Ixodes dammini* (Acari: Ixodidae). Annals of the Entomological Society of America 78:172–176.

Wilson, M. L., A. M. Ducey, T. S. Litwin, T. A. Gavin, and A. Spielman. 1990. Microgeographic distribution of immature *Ixodes dammini* ticks correlated with that of deer. Medical and Veterinary Entomology 4:151–159.

Wilson, M. L., J. F. Levine, and A. Spielman. 1984. Effect of deer reduction on abundance of the deer tick (*Ixodes dammini*). Yale Journal of Biology and Medicine 57:697–705.

Wilson, M. L., S. R. Telford, III, J. Piesman, and A. Spielman. 1988. Reduced abundance of immature *Ixodes dammini* (Acari: Ixodidae) following elimination of deer. Journal of Medical Entomology 25:224–228.

Wolff, J., and P. W. Sherman. 2007. Rodent Societies: An Ecological and Evolutionary Perspective. University of Chicago Press, Chicago.

World Health Organization. 1991. Joint WHO/FAO/UNEP panel of experts on environmental management for vector control. Geneva: World Health Organization. 80 pages. Available: http://whqlibdoc.who.int/HQ/1995/WHO_EOS_95.13.pdf

World Health Organization. 2008. World Malaria Report 2008. WHO Press, Geneva. Available: www.who.int/malaria/publications/atoz/9789241563697/en/index.html

World Health Organization Expert Committee. 2002. Prevention and Control of Schistosomiasis and Soil-Transmitted Helminthiasis. WHO Technical Report Series, no. 912.

World Health Organization, Geneva. Available: whqlibdoc.who.int/trs/WHO_
TRS_912.pdf)

Wu, D. L., C. C. Tu, C. Xin, H. Xuan, Q. W. Meng, Y. G. Liu, Y. D. Yu, Y. T. Guan, Y. Jiang,
X. N. Yin, G. Crameri, M. P. Wang, C. W. Li, S. W. Liu, M. Liao, L. Feng, H. Xiang, J.
F. Sun, J. D. Chen, Y. W. Sun, S. L. Gu, N. H. Liu, D. X. Fu, B. T. Eaton, L. F. Wang,
and X. G. Kong. 2005. Civets are equally susceptible to experimental infection by two
different severe acute respiratory syndrome coronavirus isolates. Journal of Virology
79:2620–2625.

Yates, T. L., J. N. Mills, C. A. Parmenter, T. G. Ksiazek, R. R. Parmenter, J. R. Vande Castle,
C. H. Calisher, S. T. Nichol, K. D. Abbott, J. C. Young, M. L. Morrison, B. J. Beaty, J.
L. Dunnum, R. J. Baker, J. Salazar-Bravo, and C. J. Peters. 2002. The ecology and evolutionary history of an emergent disease: hantavirus pulmonary syndrome. Bioscience
52:989–998.

Zeidner, N., M. L. Mbow, M. Dolan, R. Massung, E. Baca, and J. Piesman. 1997. Effects of
Ixodes scapularis and *Borrelia burgdorferi* on modulation of the host immune response:
induction of a TH2 cytokine response in Lyme disease-susceptible (C3H/HeJ) mice
but not in disease-resistant (BALB/c) mice. Infection and Immunity 65:3100–3106.

Zhioua, E., K. Heyer, M. Browning, H. S. Ginsberg, and R. A. LeBrun. 1999. Pathogenicity
of *Bacillus thuringiensis* variety kurstaki to *Ixodes scapularis* (Acari: Ixodidae). Journal
of Medical Entomology 36:900–902.

Zhioua, E., R. A. Lebrun, H. S. Ginsberg, and A. Aeschlimann. 1995. Pathogenicity of *Stein-
ernema carpocapsae* and *S glaseri* (Nematoda: Steinernematidae) to *Ixodes scapularis*
(Acari: Ixodidae). Journal of Medical Entomology 32:900–905.

Zhu, Y. Y., H. R. Chen, J. H. Fan, Y. Y. Wang, Y. Li, J. B. Chen, J. X. Fan, S. S. Yang, L. P.
Hu, H. Leung, T. W. Mew, P. S. Teng, Z. H. Wang, and C. C. Mundt. 2000. Genetic
diversity and disease control in rice. Nature 406:718–722.

Index

Page numbers followed by *f* denote illustrations.